MACROBIOTICS FOR EVERYONE

Other Health Books by Roger Mason

MACROBIOTICS FOR EVERYONE

A PRACTICAL & DELICIOUS APPROACH TO EATING RIGHT
FOR BETTER HEALTH, NATURAL BALANCE, AND LESS STRESS

ROGER MASON

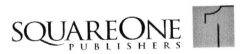

SQUAREONE
PUBLISHERS

Macrobiotics for Everyone is not intended as medical advice. It is written solely for informational and educational purposes. Please consult a health professional should the need for one be indicated. Because there are always some risks involved, the author and publisher are not responsible for any adverse affects or consequences resulting from the use of any of the suggestions, preparations, or methods described in the book. The publisher does not advocate the use of any particular diet or health program, but believes the information presented in this book should be available to the public.

All listed addresses, phone numbers, and fees have been reviewed and updated during production. However, the data is subject to change.

EDITOR: Erica Shur
COVER DESIGNER: Jeannie Tudor
TYPESETTER: Gary A. Rosenberg

Square One Publishers
115 Herricks Road
Garden City Park, NY 11040
(516) 535-2010 • (877) 900-BOOK
www.squareonepublishers.com

Library of Congress Cataloging-in-Publication Data

Mason, Roger, 1946-
  Macrobiotics for everyone : a practical & delicious approach to eating right
for better health, natural balance, and less stress / Roger Mason.
      pages cm
  1. Macrobiotic diet. 2. Diet—Religious aspects—Zen Buddhism. 3.
Meditation—Zen Buddhism. 4. Pets—Nutrition. I. Title.
  RM235.M352 2013
  613.2'64—dc23

                        2013017871

Contents

Introduction

George Ohsawa, a philosopher and writer, came to the United States in the early sixties and brought us the macrobiotic diet and lifestyle. Macrobiotics is a philosophy and a holistic approach that stresses the importance of proper dietary and lifestyle habits. For many years, it was clear that all the books on this subject were heavily influenced by Japanese culture, written by Japanese people (or with their outlook) and featuring Japanese cooking and Japanese ingredients. It became apparent there was a need for a book making macrobiotics more practical, more universal, more down to earth, more fun, tastier, more creative, sexier, less restrictive, more appealing, and without all the Japanese clothing. This book provides us with all this, without watering macrobiotics down or weakening it. There were just too many unneeded limitations, and too much cultural influence that simply did not translate. Why use expensive, hard-to-find Japanese vegetables, few soups, tea with caffeine (bancha), buckwheat noodles with white flour, refined couscous, no salads, very limited seasonings and condiments, few fresh green and yellow vegetables, all that salt, no supplements, no natural hormones, almost no raw foods, and no fasting? This book is for all cultures around the world.

There are so many natural health books today about the right foods to eat, and so many contradictory philosophies. How can one know what is valid and what is not? So many authors are very convincing. The answer is very simple—*results*. The macrobiotic way of eating is the only proven way of curing "incurable" illnesses such as the various cancers, diabetes, heart and artery problems, arthritis, osteoporosis, and the wide variety of illnesses that plague modern society, especially in the developed nations.

You have to experience this for yourself. Nature is the greatest healer, and our diet and lifestyle will allow Nature to heal us. If we are in harmony with the Natural Order, we will be healthy and happy. If we are ignorant of the Natural Order, we will be sickly and unhappy. Buddha said ignorance (to ignore), not sin, is the root cause of suffering. This is simple, clear, practical, and realistic.

We are literally what we eat. Diet causes illness, and diet cures illness. *We must take responsibility for our health, and our very destiny.* We must treat the *cause* of our illness, whether this is mental, emotional, physical, or spiritual, and not just try to remove the symptom. You cannot cure yourself by being butchered, poisoned, and irradiated. Make better food choices, take proven supplements, balance your hormones, fast weekly, end any bad habits, and exercise. This is what natural health is all about.

1. What Is Macrobiotics?

The macrobiotic way of living is based on being in harmony with the Universal Order by eating well and living well. The word "macrobiotic" comes from the Greek words "macro," or great, and "bios," or life. Hippocrates (the Father of Medicine) and Herodotus used this way of eating natural foods to regain health and to treat their patients. This way of eating was popularized in Europe and America in the 1960s, especially among younger people. George Ohsawa was the main source of information, with his rather basic books *Zen Macrobiotics* and *You Are All Sanpaku*. William Dufty and his book *Sugar Blues* were also popular. Then along came Michio Kushi, Herman Aihara, and other writers. These few authors had an immense influence, which is still strong today simply because this method of healing works. Their claims that you could cure cancer and other terminal illnesses with diet and lifestyle proved to be true. Real world experience over the decades have shown it to work. One can certainly wonder how a poor immigrant like George Ohsawa showed up here in America with no money, no credentials, or anything but his dream, yet could have such a tremendous influence on American society. Four decades later, and long after his death, macrobiotics is stronger than ever. There is an old saying: "One man plus truth equals an army." This is how George did it; he was merely a messenger with a vital, life-changing message that people here were ready to receive. His little paperback books became more and more popular. People found they made sense, and the advice really worked. Those who changed their way of eating, and their way of life, got the results he promised. They cured their illnesses by changing their direction and very destiny.

MACROBIOTIC THEORY

The underlying theory of macrobiotics is really very simple. The essence of all this is *simplicity*. Thoreau said, "Simplify, simplify, simplify." Macrobiotic principles can be adapted to all the areas of our life, and they advocate that one should rely on the body's natural ability to heal itself of illness. Allow the powers of the universe to heal you.

Diet

In current Western religions, dietetic principles are almost ignored completely. Some Seventh Day Adventists, Buddhist, and Hindu sects still observe some of them. Even the Catholics have given up abstaining from meat on Fridays. Kosher and halal foods are not based on health principles. In original Christianity, such principles were integral. In Japan today, this type of eating is called *shojin ryori*, and is still popular in the countryside (but generally not the city). Our biology and physiology are ignored instead of cared for. The teachings of the ancient religions always taught *the body is a holy temple of the spirit.* These teachings exhibit the importance of healthful eating and drinking, as well as avoiding harmful practices like coffee, tobacco, alcohol, desserts, and prescription drugs. The Code of Manu, the Bible, Canon of the Yellow Emperor, I Ching, Tao Te Ching, Bhagavad Gita, and Charak Samhita all speak of taking care of our earthly abode of consciousness, our physical body. You must be your own doctor, you must take responsibility for your health and happiness, and you must heal yourself when ill. Only you can heal yourself. "Physician, heal thyself." Be your own doctor! *Be responsible for your life.* Japanese macrobiotics overstressed whole grains. The traditional classification was seven levels of eating. One hundred percent whole grains were at the top. The lowest level was 40 percent grains. The idea of eating only whole grains as the ultimate diet is obviously unrealistic, and unhealthful for several reasons. No one can eat diet #7 (a diet that advocates eating only brown rice with a little sesame salt for a period of days, weeks, and sometimes months) with 100 percent whole grains for any length of time. You could only eat such a diet very temporarily, to heal and cleanse yourself. Such a regimen is seriously lacking in vitamins (especially vitamins A and D), minerals, and plant nutrients such as sterols and lignans. Only 50 to 60 percent of our diet should be whole grains as our principal food. Dried beans are included with grains for simplicity, and because they are so close as principal foods. Soup should consist of whole grains and beans, along with vegetables in any combination. In Japanese macrobiotics, only 5 percent was allowed to be soup, but no realistic explanation for such a limitation was given. A daily bowl of hot fla-vorful soup before dinner (and lunch as well) allows you to eat less food and feel full on fewer calories. Soups are no different from regular food, as long as you carefully chew the solids in your soup, and do not swallow unchewed food. Therefore, a very ideal and practical diet for most people would be about 50 percent whole grains and beans, 30 percent vegetables, 10 percent seafood, and 10 percent salads and/or fruits. A practical diet for the vegetarian would be about 50 percent grains and beans, 30 percent veg-etables, 10 percent salads, and 10 percent fruits. These two diets would basi-cally suit everyone, and would, in fact, cure so-called "incurable" illnesses such as cancer. Seafood should be limited to 10 percent. You can eat 10 per-cent fresh salad regularly as long as you use a light and healthy dressing. You can eat up to 10 percent local fruit, especially in the summer, but you really don't need fruit at all, especially in winter. You'll see why this is true in Chapter 7. Macrobiotic desserts are a temporary transition and an occa-sional treat, not a regular part of your diet. Desserts are really unnecessary, a Western custom, and not part of a healthy lifestyle, even if made with honey, agave, fruit juice, maple syrup, amazake, or other natural sweeten-ers. As a transition, you can temporarily make desserts out of whole grains and whole fruits with no other sweeteners. Ohsawa always made a point that *one should never waste food,* not even a single grain of rice. This may sound obsessive, but there is an important principle here. You should always eat all the food you put on your plate with great thankfulness and appreciation. Literally eat the last grain of rice on your plate to show respect for the Universal Order. One never wastes food.

As part of a macrobiotic diet, one eats whole grains as the main, prin-cipal food. Beans and legumes are also staples. Most green and yellow veg-etables are used. Soups, salads, and local fruit are eaten in moderation. Seafood can be eaten in moderation, or you can choose to be a vegetarian. Tropical foods from hot climates, such as bananas, citrus fruit, and mangoes are avoided for those living in temperate climates, regardless of their genet-ic inheritance. You should avoid nightshade vegetables, including potatoes, tomatoes, peppers, and eggplants, as they contain large amounts of toxic solanine. Tomatoes also contain toxic tomatine. Also, avoid vegetables high in oxalic acid, such as spinach and Swiss chard. People living in a temper-ate climate people should avoid tropical vegetables such as taro root, boni-ata, yucca, etc. This is discussed in Chapter 6. The most important food to eliminate is milk and dairy foods, due to their lactose and casein content. All adults of all races are lactose intolerant. Casein promotes cancer and other diseases. Everyone loses their ability to secrete the enzyme lactase after about three years of age. Red meat is too full of saturated fat and cholesterol. Poultry and eggs are high in saturated fat, and are two of the most allergenic of all foods. Basically, sweeteners are not used, including honey and maple syrup. Just because a food is "natural" does not mean it is healthful and suited for us to eat. There are many natural foods that do not support a long and healthy life. One drinks good well or filtered water or herbal tea, and eats only two meals a day. No meat, milk, dairy products, poultry, or eggs are eaten. If one wants to be a vegetarian, then seafood is left out. One always adapts to one's genetics, the climate, and the seasons. This, simply put, is what comprises the macrobiotic way of eating. This way of eating is always adaptable and flexible for each person.

Lifestyle

Happy societies are based on millions of happy individuals. Imagine if the almost 7 billion people on this earth ate and drank and lived in harmony with the Divine Order. This planet would be all we have dreamed of, and more. Our health and happiness are determined by our judgment, by our awareness, and by our faith in the Infinite. With good judgment we can be happy and healthy. Macrobiotics is based on clear judgment, and there are no rigid rules to follow. There are principles to lead us, but no dogma we must obey. Instead of structure, there is flow. As the Zen master Lin-Chi said, "At one stroke I forgot all my knowledge! There is no need for any discipline, for, move as I will, I always manifest the Tao." Macrobiotics is a deep understanding of the Ultimate Ground of Being that underlies our very existence. Above all, this is practical, pragmatic, logical, rational, sensible, based on common sense, and relates to the most everyday and mundane aspects of our lives. This includes washing the dishes and driving to work. We come to realize the Divine in the everyday, not some other world. The more we understand the Order of the Universe, the more we harmonize with it, and eat the foods that are best for us. As artists we create our own lives and design our own lifestyles by living in harmony with universal laws. Design your life! We become our own doctors, and follow the admonition "Physician, heal thyself." As we become more aware, we gain freedom, health, happiness, creativity, and spiritual realization. We take full and total responsibility for our lives, and do not blame conditions, circumstances, or other people for our faults, limitations, problems, and unhappiness. Look at your life…are you happy with it? *Your life is exactly the way you made it* and you are free to change it any way you choose in your heart. Do you love it? Do you hate it? There it is, the way you made it! In your innermost being, do you really want to be a famous actor or actress, a powerful and influential politician, a billionaire business magnate, or a legendary sports figure? These are empty, meaningless, and narcissistic fantasies. Do such people find *true* happiness and fulfillment? Our overall attitude should be one of *thankfulness,* and being grateful for all we have been given, not taking anything for granted. We should always be thankful just for being incarnated in physical bodies, and being on this earth. It is very rare to be given the gift of being alive in human form. Life is a brief flash of light in the cosmos, and we have been given this chance to live any way we want to, and to be anything we want to be. Always be thankful and grateful simply for being alive on this earth as a sentient, aware being. We all manifest the entire universe. We are all microcosms of the Infinite Universe. We are powerful spiritual beings.

CONCLUSION

Our environment, genetics, what we choose to eat and drink, and how we live our lives determines our destiny, our health, and who we are. The macrobiotic life stresses a proper dietary regimen and lifestyle routine, both of which will be discussed throughout the book. You will come to greatly enjoy grains, beans, vegetables, seafood, soups, salads, and fruits. You will soon not miss the meat, poultry, eggs, dairy foods, refined foods, and sugars that Americans eat so much of. This will become a natural and fulfilling way of life for you. As well as dietary changes, macrobiotics inspires one to make lifestyle and environmental changes.

2. Yin and Yang

No book on macrobiotics would be complete without talking about yin and yang. In Taoist philosophy, yin and yang is the unifying principle where the interplay of opposites is central. Yin is the feminine, cold, contracting, violet energy, while yang is the masculine, hot, and expanding red energy. Together, the universe, and everything in it, is made, preserved, and dissolved. The universe we live in is not solid at all, as we think, but rather an energy dance of vibrations. Existence is without beginning or end, beyond space and time, and ever changing. Yin and yang are relative terms, and not absolutes. Everything has both forces in it, and nothing is purely yin or purely yang. The most yang substance has yin at its heart, while the most yin substance has yang at its heart. Yin and yang are a celestial dance. Ohsawa called this "our guiding compass." Using this principle shows us the right direction in our daily lives.

THE CLASSIFICATIONS
OF YIN AND YANG

A very good way to look at the foods we eat is that a balance of yin and yang forces should prevail. Too much yin, or too much yang, ends up in sickness and ill health. You cannot balance yin and yang by going to extremes. Eating a very yin food, like candy, and then eating a very yang food, like beef, will not create balance. You cannot cook tomatoes (yin) with salt (yang) to make them less yin; the chemical constitution will remain the same, basically. Balance means to eat proper foods in the right amounts, so that a natural equilibrium prevails. How does this apply to what we eat? The most yin foods to yang foods goes from yin drugs (e.g. stimulants) → sugars → alcohol → yeast → oil → fruit → yin dairy (e.g. yogurt) → nuts → water → green and yellow vegetables → sea vegetables → beans → grains → seafood → yang dairy (e.g. hard cheese) → poultry → meat → eggs → salt → yang drugs (e.g. opiates). Dairy products can be yin like yogurt, or yang like hard cheese. Drugs can be yin like stimulants, or yang like opiates. Please look at this chain of food very carefully, from yin to yang, and remember it. You can see that vegetables, beans, and grains are the basis of our diet. This gives you an idea of how to avoid the extremes, to balance your body, mind, health, and life. You cannot stay healthy by eating, for example, honey and fish, and expecting them to balance each other out. You can see in our present society that poor health comes largely from an extreme intake of sweeteners of various types on one hand and extreme intake of animal products on the other hand. The yin and yang classification is very helpful with colors as well. Colors go from yin ultraviolet → violet → indigo-blue → green → yellow → brown → orange → red yang infrared.

You can take this too far, however. The original Japanese writers certainly did. In the real world, this only works to a certain degree, and then becomes too complex for it to be practical anymore. A perfect example is cherry tomatoes. These are small (yang), round (yang), and red (yang), but are one of the top ten allergenic foods on earth, and chemically very yin. Whether you eat big, pear-shaped, yellow tomatoes or little, round cherry red tomatoes makes no real difference. Most all people are biologically incompatible with them, and will react negatively to their regular intake. Too much concern about what is yin and what is yang, and how to make yin foods more yang, and yang foods more yin, becomes more like arguing about how many angels can dance on the head of a pin than eating a balanced diet!

THE PRINCIPLES
OF YIN AND YANG

Yin and yang are the essential principles of Chinese philosophy. The fundamental doctrine of the concepts is that everything is part of a whole. The equilibrium between yin and yang can explain relationships, patterns, and changes. Some things to remember:

Yin and yang are always relative.
Whatever has a beginning has an end.
No two things are identical.

Oneness always manifests itself at all times as two forces.
> Yin and yang are always changing into each other.
> Yin attracts yang, and yang attracts yin.
> Yin repels yin, and yang repels yang.

Nothing is only yin or only yang; everything is composed of both yin and yang together.

Nothing is balanced and static; everything is made up of dynamic and unequal portions of yin and yang.
> The bigger the front, the bigger the back.
> The bigger the problem, the bigger the opportunity.
> All antagonisms are, in reality, complementary.

The entire universe is unchanging, limitless, infinite, constant, and omnipotent. There are no mistakes.

Your worst enemy is your best friend, and will teach you more than anyone else.

Every experience in your life is exactly what you need at that moment, and must be learned, or it will be repeated. There are no mistakes in the universe. Everything is exactly the way it is supposed to be.

CONCLUSION

The philosophy of yin and yang tells us that all things are always balancing and rebalancing into a state of perfect harmony. It is a way of life that stresses living harmoniously with nature, and eating and living in harmony with universal laws. The macrobiotic diet and way of life allows us to enjoy life to the fullest and realize our inner nature. The following chapters will outline the locally grown foods that will satisfy this balance.

3. Whole Grains

Whole *grains are literally the staff of life.* Whole grains have been the staple of most civilizations since man mastered the art of agriculture over ten thousand years ago. The word "cereal" comes from the goddess Ceres. When man learned how to grow his own food, and not merely hunt and gather, he gained freedom for the first time. This was the major defining difference between cave people, at the mercy of natural forces, and those who forged their own destiny. Americans and Europeans no longer eat many whole grains, however, and haven't for a long time. They eat a mere one percent. The rice is white, the bread is white, the cornmeal is degermed, the cold cereal is refined, and the flour is white. We have almost forgotten about such wonderful foods like oats, barley, buckwheat, and millet. Why base your diet on whole grains? This has been the staple food for mankind for thousands of years, and rightly so. Let's use extremes to make a point. If you ate nothing but red meat for a month, what effects would it have? You would suffer from ketosis (high blood ketones), high cholesterol and triglycerides, elevated uric acid, bad body and mouth odor, a general feeling of malaise, physical weakness, and other problems. What if you ate only fruit for one month? The effects would be extremely disrupted blood glucose metabolism, severe lack of nutrition, and a dangerous sugar overload. Consuming only eggs and poultry would lead to very similar effects as consuming only meat, but worse, since so many people have allergies to poultry and eggs. What about only eating green and yellow vegetables? You would lose weight and lack protein and other nutrients, but would certainly feel good and look better. You could not continue on such a regimen, though. Whole grains? You would feel and look wonderful, your mind would be clear, you would be full of energy, your body would be cleansed, your body fat would fall, and many illnesses and conditions would be healed. Long term, you would lack certain vitamins (especially vitamin A), minerals, and other nutrients that are found in beans and green and yellow vegetables. Clearly whole grains are our principal food.

Let's take one specific example as proof. What is the most rapidly growing epidemic in the world by far? Diabetes and other blood sugar disorders are the worst health threat we face. One in three American children will grow up to suffer from type 2 diabetes! People who eat the most whole grains have the lowest rates of diabetes. People who eat the least whole grains have the highest rates. Do we have published clinical proof this is true? Yes, there is overwhelming evidence of this. Our own United States Department of Agriculture states this. The University of Minnesota proved this in studying over 160,000 men and women. The National Public Health Institute of Finland proved this is true. Harvard Medical School has published several studies on this. The most impressive of all is the Framingham Study, which is the longest and largest ongoing study of diet and health. Since this is true for diabetes, it is certainly equally true for coronary heart disease—our biggest killer by far—various cancers, and the other disease conditions we suffer from.

WHOLE GRAINS

We eat twice the protein we need, five times the fat, as well as twice the calories. The reality is that protein deficiency rarely ever exists, but protein overload is an epidemic. The average whole grain contains about 8 percent high quality protein. This is readily bioavailable with a wide variety of amino acids. When you eat beans regularly you will have an even larger variety of amino acids. The idea of lacking certain amino acids, and having "incomplete" proteins, is not based on science at all. You will get plenty of complete protein on a macrobiotic diet, even if you choose to be a vegetarian and eat no seafood. Gluten intolerance is almost nonexistent. The only basic grains to even contain gluten are wheat, rye, and barley.

Wheat

Let's start with wheat. Nearly all the wheat eaten in America is in the form of refined white flour. Even the "whole wheat" bread in the grocery stores is usually adulterated with white flour, chemicals, and preservatives, as well as being too light and fluffy. Most bakeries do not sell real whole wheat bread, but rather "wheat bread" with unbleached white flour added. Buy your bread from a natural food store, a bakery that sells the real thing, or make it yourself. Whole wheat breads vary quite a bit according to weight, water content, slice thickness, and even the amount of oil added. A typical slice has about 70 calories and 13 percent fat calories. Most all the various pastas are made from white flour, or a mixture of white and whole wheat flours. You can readily find a wide variety of whole wheat pasta now in most chain grocery stores. Two ounces of dry whole wheat spaghetti is about 200 calories. When cooked al dente, this is only about 5 percent fat calories, and will weigh about six ounces, drained. Bulgur wheat is whole wheat that has been soaked to expand it, and then dried, so it cooks more quickly. This retains most of the whole grain nutrition, contains only about 152 calories per cup cooked, and a mere 3 percent fat calories. Bulgur is not well known. Regular couscous is nearly always a refined grain, and should only be eaten occasionally in Middle Eastern restaurants. Look for whole wheat couscous in natural health food stores for regular use. Whole wheat tortillas are best made at home with a simple ten dollar tortilla press. Good ones are difficult to find, even in Latino grocery stores. Commercial cold cereals are rarely made with whole wheat. The few that are, have sugar added to them. Fortunately, you can now find a few good whole grain cold cereals in chain groceries, and not just natural food stores. A typical brand has only about 120 calories per cup (30 g) dry. You'll rarely find whole wheat products when you go out to eat in restaurants. Yes, there are occasional uses for unbleached white flour at times as a thickener in white sauces and soups, but not to replace whole wheat flour in breads and such.

It is true you should eat more steamed grains, rather than flour products like bread, and noodles. Steamed whole grains retain more nutrition than pasta, bread, and other flour products. Traditional macrobiotics recommends sourdough bread, as if this is somehow not leavened with yeast. All risen bread is still based on yeast, wild or otherwise. About the only unleavened bread is matzoh. Yes, yeast is very yin, but it is completely dead after baking. You are getting very little cooked yeast protein in a slice of bread. You should look for heavy, dense loaves that weigh about two pounds, and are about eight inches long and four inches high.

Whole unprocessed grains have a long shelf life, while retaining their nutrition. Once ground into flour, however, they oxidize and lose their valuable nutrients. Ideally you should grind your own flour, but this is not practical for most people. It is best to buy refrigerated, fresh-ground whole wheat bread or pastry (low gluten) flour in a natural food store if possible. You will find different uses for both bread and pastry flours. If you can't grind your own, then buy your flour in the grocery store and keep it refrigerated. The reason white flour does not need to be refrigerated is that the oils and nutrients have been refined out of it. Definitely, you want to eat more steamed grains than flour products (such as noodles and bread) as a general rule.

Brown Rice

Brown rice is sold in most groceries now. Some Asian restaurants, especially in big cities like New York or Los Angeles, offer brown rice with your meal if you request it. It is worthwhile buying 25 pound bags of organically grown brown rice, since many chemicals are used to raise regular rice. You can buy exotic brown rice like jasmine and basmati if you're willing to pay up for them. The short-grain variety is usually preferred, as it is supposedly more yang. It really makes little difference. It is worth the price to get organically grown rice, since it will be your staple. You can also find short-grain sweet rice, but this takes longer to cook correctly, and is really meant for desserts rather than meals. Brown rice pasta is popular now, but you have to cook it carefully, never cook it too long, and cool it off once it is finished. Brown rice flour is available, and mostly used for baking. You can readily find brown rice hot and cold cereals. These usually use brown rice in a mix with other whole grains. Rice is most versatile, and can be used in many ways in very different types of dishes. A lot of people choose to eat brown rice as their staple food. They feel it simply tastes better than the other grains. One cup of cooked brown rice has about 173 calories and 5 percent fat calories. People in Japan, Thailand, Korea, Vietnam, and China generally eat white rice.

Wild Rice

Wild rice, like buckwheat, is not botanically classed as a grain. Wild rice is really a grass with a strong flavor. It is pricey when compared to brown rice. This is a perfectly good food, but you may want to use it to flavor your brown rice and other grains, rather than eat it by itself. The taste is simply too assertive. This makes a good addition to your other grains, and adds variety and flavor. It has even fewer calories than brown rice, as it contains only 3 percent fat calories.

Corn

Corn is still eaten whole as a vegetable, as corn on the cob. Frozen corn is acceptable out of season. White or yellow cornmeal is popular, but make sure it is whole, and not "degermed," with the nutrition removed. A fancy word for cornmeal mush is polenta. This is served in some of the finest restaurants, especially Northern Italian ones. If you have never had polenta, it is very easy and quick to fix, quite good, and inexpensive. Just take one cup of cornmeal and three cups of water or vegetable stock, and cook for about fifteen minutes. You can replace one cup of stock with nondairy milk to make it creamy. Corn grits are a Southern staple, but have been degermed, and are not a whole grain. Even Mexican white hominy (maiz trillado) is degermed. It seems that whole corn grits do not exist for some reason. Anything labeled "hominy" is usually degermed corn, unfortunately. Good corn chips that are baked rather than fried can be an excellent whole grain food. Latins use masa harina, or finely ground corn flour, rather than coarse meal. Be sure this is ground from whole corn, and not degermed. An ear of corn has about 89 calories with 10 percent fat calories, and is equal to a half cup of fresh or frozen corn kernels. A quarter cup of whole cornmeal (30 g) has 100 calories and 10 percent fat calories. Cooked with three quarters of a cup of water, or stock, this would make a large serving of polenta. You can find special coarse ground meal labeled as such.

Oats

Oats are rarely eaten now, except as oatmeal for breakfast. Too often this is instant or quick-cooking. Be sure to buy the old-fashioned oatmeal, as it still cooks quickly. Oat groats and steel cut oats are other good choices. Very few people use oat flour, but it goes well in breads and baking. Oat flakes also go very well in baking. Some whole grain cold cereals include oats in them. This is a yang cereal with high oil content. It grows in cold regions, and is very good for cold climates and in winter time. A cup of cooked oatmeal has 145 calories and 12 percent fat calories, so it is especially good for cold weather. It's a shame such a fine, flavorful grain is now generally limited only to breakfast cereal. Oats also are a wonderful source of beta glucan for your immunity. Oats contain huge amounts (5 percent dry weight) of beta glucan. A mere ounce has 1,400 mg!

Buckwheat

Buckwheat is not botanically a grain, but certainly is rightly considered a grain for practical purposes. You can buy buckwheat groats in the grocery store. Very few people eat buckwheat groats anymore, but they are quite good and mix well with other grains. Try half buckwheat and half brown rice for a change. Buckwheat cooks very easily and quickly. You can find hot cereals made with buckwheat as well. An emphasis was made in macrobiotics about eating buckwheat noodles, or soba. At Asian stores you will find that all the buckwheat noodles are filled with white flour. Buckwheat lacks gluten to hold it together, and must be mixed with wheat flour. It is difficult to find buckwheat noodles made with whole wheat flour for some reason. When found, they are very expensive, and simply have no advantage over whole wheat pastas. Buckwheat groats are delicious, can be mixed with other grains, and are very nutritious. This is especially good in winter since they are very yang and grown in cold climates such as Canada.

Rye

Rye is not commonly eaten today, except mixed with white flour in rye bread. Nearly all rye is used to make whiskey. Rye has a strong and distinctive flavor, so it should not be used alone in bread. There are a few hot cereals made with rye, but they are not very widely sold. When you make your own whole grain bread, be sure to make some rye bread occasionally. Use one-third rye and two-thirds whole wheat flour, along with caraway seeds and cornmeal.

Millet

Millet is a popular staple in some African countries, but not very popular here. You can buy whole millet and discover a whole new grain to eat. It is easy to find and inexpensive. This cooks quickly, and can be mixed with your rice for variety. You can add millet flour to homemade bread as well. You'll find this in multigrain breads often. A cup of cooked millet contains about 287 calories and 6 percent fat calories. This seems high because cooked millet does not contain much water and is very filling. It is a fine grain to eat, with a lot of nutrition.

Barley

Barley is mostly used in soup, but can be used just like brown rice. It is also a wonderful source of beta glucan for your immunity, and like oats, contains huge amounts (5 percent dry weight) of beta glucan. Most all barley is pearled, as the hull is inedible. One cup of cooked barley contains about 193 calories and only 6 percent fat calories.

Other Grains

What about spelt, teff, triticale, and quinoa? These are ancient grains, and can be hard to find, and rather expensive, compared to other grains. Try these for variety, as they do differ in taste. You will find baked goods and pastas containing these. As they become more common, the price will come down. Some grains can be successfully sprouted, including barley, buckwheat, rice, wheat, millet, oats, and triticale. You can find these in natural food stores or easily sprout them at home. Treat sprouts as vegetables, since that is what they are nutritionally after being sprouted.

Get some cookbooks on how to cook grains in a variety of international styles. You'll find they quickly become an immensely enjoyable principal food you look forward to every day. It can be difficult at first to use whole grains as your principal food when you haven't been used to them. Once you learn to cook them, they will become the main course of your every meal. You'll come to love whole grains as the center of your diet and look forward to enjoying them in a variety of ways.

CONCLUSION

If you could eat only one food to stay alive temporarily during an emergency, your best choice would be to pick any whole grain. You could thrive on this for a long time. *Whole grains are your staple food*, and should be the basis of your diet, your principal food. Whole grains are easily digested, and leave no toxins in the body during their metabolism. They contain all the protein you need, are very low in fat, high in fiber, low in calories, and very concentrated in nutrition. Whole grains are also the best food to regulate your blood sugar. Blood sugar dysmetabolism is epidemic in Western societies, largely because we have forgotten whole grains as our main source of nutrition. This is the central food of the macrobiotic way of eating.

4. Beans
Are Good Food

Beans and legumes are wonderful foods that feed much of the world. Beans are very high in protein, vitamins, minerals, and plant nutrients like lignans and sterols, but without the calories or the fat. People who begin eating beans regularly sometimes have excess gas or bloating. This basically goes away as the body gets acclimated to eating them and your intestines become healthier. There are digestive enzymes such as alpha galactosidase, also known as Beano, which are available if you want to take them, but it isn't necessary. Dried beans should also be a staple in your diet. You will come to enjoy them very much, as you learn to cook and flavor them in international styles. In affluent societies such as ours, they are often looked at as food for poor people.

TYPES OF BEANS

Characteristically rich in both fiber and protein, low-fat beans (legumes) are the mainstays of a macrobiotic diet. Beans are packed with vitamins, minerals, and essential nutrients, and have been perfect staples for a healthy diet. Different beans have different healing powers. The different types of beans and their nutritional value provide us with some of the best ways to obtain our quota of lean protein and fiber. Your local supermarket or food stores stock a wide variety of beans and legumes such as pintos, lentils, black-eyed peas, chili beans, black beans, northern, pink, chickpeas, kidneys, limas, navy, and cannellini beans. Rarer beans can be found at a Latin market, and here you'll find beans you've probably never heard of. Buy one of each variety, like pigeon peas and favas, and go home and try them. At gourmet stores or on the Internet, you'll really find some interesting beans, such as appaloosa, calypso, Christmas limas, cranberry, European soldiers, yellow eyed peas, white emergo, trout, tongues of fire, Swedish brown beans, snow-caps, scarlet runners, Spanish tolosanas, French flageolets, French navy, Jackson wonders, piebald, Provence, rattlesnake, rice, and other international beans.

TABLE 4.1 NUTRITIONAL PROFILE OF COMMON BEANS (PER HALF CUP COOKED)			
Bean (half cup cooked)	Calories	Percent Fat	Percent Protein
Chickpeas	120	4	20
Kidney	112	1	20
Lentils	115	1	26
Pinto/Calico	117	1	19
Lima	111	1	20
Black-eyed	100	2	17
Yellow soybeans	139	14	29
Red beans	100	1	20
Black beans	113	4	23
Navy bean	129	1	21
Northern beans	104	1	19
Pink beans	125	1	20
Cannellini	125	1	20
Fava (Broad)	100	2	30
Split peas	115	1	24
Mayacabo	81	0	25

COOKING WITH BEANS

At libraries or bookstores you can locate international cookbooks and see how the cooks of the world prepare their beans. Bean soups, refried beans, pasta and beans, bean dips, bean salads, and bean spreads like hummus, show their versatility. Some beans can be sprouted, especially soy, mung, lentil, green and yellow peas, chickpeas, and adzuki beans. Try adding bean thread to your soups and stir fries. The early macrobiotic teachers emphasized adzuki beans, only because the Japanese actually eat very few beans in their diet. Enjoy all varieties of beans cooked in various international styles with good herbal flavorings.

It can take 2 to 3 hours to cook beans, so you can cook up a pound bag, and freeze half of them if you want to. Remember to bring them to a boil, turn off the heat, and let them hot soak for a few hours before cooking. Do not add salt until after they have fully soaked. Never add baking soda to make them cook quicker, as some cookbooks suggest. Adding vegetables such as garlic, carrots, onions, leeks, and celery, makes beans more flavorful, nutritious, colorful, and interesting. Be sure to use your favorite herbs, spices, and flavorings to make them even more delicious.

TOFU

What about tofu, which is so popular? Tofu, originating in China, is also called bean curd. This is a very versatile food, but a very refined one. Tofu is low in calories, but also very low in nutrition. It cannot be sautéed, as it absorbs oil like a sponge. It certainly does have limited uses, but this is just not a staple food. Tofu is the white bread of soybeans. Tempeh is a whole food, and a much better choice since it has all the nutrition of the soybean, low in fat and high in protein. Tempeh is firm and has a nutty flavor. It can be found in most grocery stores in their refrigerated section.

CONCLUSION

Dry beans have been consumed as a diet staple throughout history. They provide a wealth of nutrients and may help in reducing the risk of disease. However, most Americans are not eating enough beans. When you learn to use and cook beans in new and creative ways, you'll come to enjoy them as a regular part of your diet. Beans are next to grains as a principal food due to their high nutrition, good protein, high fiber, low fat content, and low calories. Beans are good food.

5. Vegetables

Most Americans are rather bored by green and yellow vegetables, basically due to the poor cooking and flavoring methods used to prepare them. Most restaurants rarely serve more than one green or yellow vegetable, except for some homestyle restaurants in the South. Fast food restaurants serve almost none. Even gourmet restaurants often only offer one single vegetable du jour. The uncreative way green and yellow vegetables are generally prepared, cooked, and served in North America is a very good reason more people are not attracted to them. Many people still buy mushy canned vegetables! Some frozen vegetables are very tasty and full of nutrition, and can be acceptable in winter when they are out of season. Fortunately, we have a wide variety of fresh vegetables available all year round here in America. Most people eat their vegetables boiled until they're soggy, and then flavored with butter, salt, and pepper. Nearly all Latin countries are the same way, and avoid green and yellow vegetables for some reason. The Asians generally are the premier vegetable cooks. The main Asian preparation is a stir fry with lots of good flavors added, such as ginger, garlic, soy sauce, sherry, oyster sauce, dark sesame oil, black bean sauce, chili sauce, and other such condiments. Get some Chinese, Vietnamese, Indonesian, and Thai cookbooks for interesting ways to fix and flavor your favorite vegetables.

TYPES OF VEGETABLES

One could easily get the idea from reading the early macrobiotic books that Diet #7 is the ideal. This diet claims that eating more grains and less vegetables is better. This is a big misunderstanding, as eating only whole grains was really suggested as a very temporary regimen for people with serious illness. It is important to eat lots of fresh green and yellow vegetables with your grains and beans. Vegetables contain vitamins and other nutrients, such as vitamin A, beta carotene, vitamin C, and sterols, which are not found in grains. You can eat as much as 50 percent fresh vegetables, and should eat at least 25 percent. You'll eat more vegetables in the summer, when you need lighter food and fewer calories, and less in the winter, when you need heavier food and more calories.

Common Vegetables

Let's take a look at some of the many good vegetables we can eat. Asparagus, artichoke, bok choy, bush and pole beans, bean sprouts, beets, broccoli, Brussels sprouts, red and green cabbage, Chinese cabbage, carrots, cauliflower, celery, Swiss chard (occasionally), cucumbers, garlic, edible gourds, endive, collards, kale, lettuce (various), mustard greens, kohlrabi, leeks, lotus root, many types of mushrooms, okra, onions, parsnips, peas, snow peas, various pumpkins, radishes, rutabagas, salsify, Malabar spinach and New Zealand spinach, green and yellow squashes, various winter squashes, green beans, sweet potatoes (which are not yams), turnips, and watercress. Vegetables contain few calories, much less than any other food group.

TABLE 5.1 CALORIE CONTENT OF COMMON VEGETABLES (PER 100 GRAMS)			
Vegetable	Calories	Vegetable	Calories
Artichoke	26	Kale	33
Asparagus	26	Leeks	52
Beets	31	Lettuce	35
Broccoli	18	Mushrooms	40
Brussels sprouts	32	Onions	24
Cabbage	27	Radishes	17
Carrots	52	Squash, Summer	14
Cauliflower	27	Squash, Winter	25
Celery	14	Turnip Greens	24
Cucumber	9		

Rare Vegetables

The older macrobiotic books also kept recommending such hard to obtain and expensive vegetables like burdock root, mountain yams (nagaimo), Hokkaido pumpkin, daikon radish, and other such Japanese foods. These just don't translate here very well. They have no advantage over the vegetables we have in America, and can be very hard to find, even in Asian food stores.

Raw Vegetables

You rarely see raw vegetables or raw salads recommended in traditional macrobiotics. It is true that people on an all raw food diet quickly become very sickly, and they have to stop such a regimen. Raw foods are part of eating well, especially in the summer, when lighter fare is needed. Most vegetables are simply inedible when eaten raw. They need light cooking to make them palatable. The old macrobiotic idea of pressing and salting your salad greens is very unnecessary and ruins crisp lettuce and other raw vegetables. A small salad makes a wonderful and colorful addition to any meal, especially in summer, when there are fewer calories consumed. The real concern is finding a low-fat or no-fat dressing to go on your salads. Many Latinos have a custom of simply squeezing lime juice over their salad, and do not use creamy dressings at all. Asians flavor their salad greens with such condiments as soy sauce, sesame, and ginger.

The entire Allium (onion) family—onions, leeks, garlic, and green onions—must always be cooked to evaporate the irritating volatile oils, and must never be eaten raw. Raw garlic and onions are used as natural insecticides due to their irritating nature. Certain yogic systems do not allow onions and garlic, as they are considered too "rajastic." (This means overly stimulating and disturbing to the body.) Some people will be allergic and biologically incompatible with the Allium family, and should not eat them. If you get indigestion from eating any of these, please drop them from your diet. It is true that the substances in garlic have been shown in countless clinical studies to have healing properties for most people. This has been verified clinically over the years, but some people will still be allergic.

Salted and Salt-Pickled Vegetables

Salted and salt-pickled vegetables are popular in cold, remote areas where produce is seasonal. This is about the only way they can obtain green and yellow vegetables in winter. The salt overload from such foods is excessive. Pickled vegetables are still popular in Asian areas where there is no refrigeration. There is just no reason to eat high sodium pickled vegetables, including such things as preserved daikon radish. It is far preferable to eat fresh or frozen vegetables, since a wide variety are available all year round. There are times when frozen vegetables are fine in winter. There is a loss of texture in these, but no loss of nutrition. Canned vegetables are generally avoided.

Sea Vegetables

Sea vegetables are commonly referred to as seaweeds. Traditional macrobiotics recommends we eat these very nutritious vegetables from the ocean, including nori, kombu, and hiziki. These are the best source of minerals we can eat, and they can be found at Asian grocery stores. Americans have never cultivated much of a taste for these. Most people refuse to eat them, except maybe as nori-wrapped sushi. Buy some of the various sea vegetables, and at least try them in small amounts. You only need a tablespoonful at meals and it makes an elegant garnish. However, there is a problem with these, in that they contain extremely high amounts of iodine. *Only use them in moderation.* Some people may react to such high doses of iodine, and should avoid them.

PREPARING VEGETABLES

When prepared well, vegetables can be quite delicious. Get some international cookbooks, and see how the chefs of the world prepare different vegetables. Modify any recipes if possible that sound good that can be made with healthy ingredients. Most recipes can be adapted to be healthful. Tempura vegetables are popular in Japanese restaurants, but are very high in oil content, no matter how skillfully cooked. This certainly tastes good, but it is not a good way to eat them regularly. Tempura is best reserved for special occasions. You can use a pressure cooker if you choose to, but very few people do. The idea that this makes food more yang is technically true, but rather unimportant. If you want to cook your grains and certain dishes in a pressure cooker, they are very safe, easy to use, and cook your food more quickly.

Note that sprouts weren't included in traditional Japanese macrobiotics. However, there are many seeds that can be sprouted to add taste and variety to your vegetables, salads, and sandwiches. Many sprouts are now available in grocery stores. Making sprouts at home is easy and fun. Some vegetable seeds that can be successfully sprouted are alfalfa, cabbage, broccoli, Brussels sprouts, cauliflower, kale, chia, cress, radish, and fenugreek.

If you want to lose weight and consume less calories, simply eat more good green and yellow vegetables. You should eat 50 percent or more whole grains as your principal food. To lose weight you can eat more green and yellow vegetables, salads, soups, local fruits, but little or no seafood. This is filling but very low calorie. When you don't feel like fasting, you can go on a vegetable soup diet for a week or two. You can lose an impressive amount of weight while never being hungry. Just make soups from your favorite grains, beans, green vegetables, and yellow vegetables. Flavor these fully. This is a partial fast and will also benefit your health from the very low calorie intake.

CONCLUSION

A natural and holistic lifestyle includes eating healthy foods, including vegetables, several servings of yellow and green vegetables, as discussed in this chapter. Although a macrobiotic diet recommends eating at least one serving of vegetables a day, if not more, it also recommends avoiding certain vegetables, like nightshades. We learn more about these nightshade vegetables in the next chapter.

6. Tropical and Nightshade Foods

The macrobiotic philosophy has always been the only dietary philosophy to warn against nightshade vegetables. Why don't other dietary proponents warn us against these? The toxic chemical constituents of these plants have been well known to scientists for over a century. Deadly nightshades are botanically known as the Solanaceae family. This includes potatoes, tomatoes (botanically a fruit), eggplants, most peppers, belladonna, Jimson weed, and tobacco. This family obviously includes dangerous and even deadly plants. These vegetables contain harmful glycoalkaloids, especially solanine, tomatine, and chaconine. Each year, the average American consumes enough solanine to kill an entire family of four—from potatoes alone. No other diets exclude the Solanaceae family, only macrobiotics.

SOLANINE FOODS

Green-skinned potatoes are especially dangerous due to the very high level of glycoalkaloids. Potato sprouts also contain very dangerous amounts. Potatoes can vary widely in toxic alkaloid content, but about 12 mg per 100-g serving is typical. Some varieties contain up to 30 mg per 100-g serving. You can eat potatoes, say, once a week, but they are unfit for regular use. All the industrialized countries seem to live off meat and potatoes. Americans, Canadians, English, Scottish, Welsh, Irish, German, French, Swiss, Austrians, Australians, and New Zealanders all love potatoes as a major dietary staple. Americans are estimated to eat over 60 kg a year, which comes to about 170 grams per day (almost 6 ounces). We eat mashed potatoes, baked potatoes, the ubiquitous French fry, hash browns, potato pancakes, potato chips, and potato salad. Why this love affair with a mere tuber, other than the fact it is inexpensive, easy to grow, and very versatile? The Asian countries did not eat potatoes until very recently and still do not embrace them.

For centuries the tomato was considered an ornamental plant unfit to eat. They are not native to the United States, and were not popular at all until about 50 years ago. We should have retained that native wisdom, and kept them for decoration. It is only recently that Americans started to eat large amounts of tomatoes and tomato products, especially canned ones. Concentrated tomato paste contains the most alkaloids. In addition to solanine, they also contain the toxic glycolalkaloid tomatine, which has similar effects. Tomatoes are one of the top ten known allergenic foods. Most people are, in fact, demonstrably allergic to them. Many people break out if they eat them. Yet, millions of tons are eaten every year in ketchup, pasta sauce, tomato juice, salads, pizza, and other foods. Southern Italy is the major country to make a cult of the tomato; the Northern Italians only use them occasionally. All the natural diet authors include tomatoes as a regular staple. They just don't understand the toxicity of these nightshade alkaloids. If you ate just one tomato a day for a year, the solanine in them would actually kill an entire family of four if ingested all at once. Just like potatoes. Yes, you certainly can put a slice of tomato on your sandwich if you like, or eat a red sauce occasionally.

Eggplants (Solanum melongena), or aubergines, are just not very popular, and never have been in America. The amount of solanine varies, but typically is about 8 mg per 100-g serving, and ranges from about 6 to 11 mg. Eggplants are just not commonly used here, and are mostly found in Italian and Thai cooking.

Peppers (Capsicum family), including bell peppers, are very popular in the United States. They also contain about 8 mg of solanine per 100-g serving. Peppers can be used occasionally in small amounts. This Capsicum family does not include black pepper, but that should be avoided for other reasons. Green bell peppers are an American staple, but should only be eaten in moderation.

OXALATE FOODS

There is another group of foods to be cautious of, and that is the oxalate group. Most common vegetables contain small amounts of oxalic acid. Some foods contain higher quantities than other vegetables, and should only be eaten occasionally. Oxalic acid binds with minerals, especially calcium and iron, to form urinary stones. Kidney stones are very common, and also due to excessive dairy intake. Vegetables such as Swiss chard, spinach, sorrel, amaranth, rhubarb, beet leaves, parsley, purslane, chives, and cassava root contain high amounts of oxalic acid. These contribute to poor health if eaten daily. These foods can be eaten occasionally in small amounts, but not regularly.

EFFECTS OF NIGHTSHADE VEGETABLES

One major reason for the existing epidemic of arthritis and rheumatism is our intake of nightshade alkaloids. These toxins actually accumulate in our tissues over time. Clinical studies have shown the effect of nightshade vegetables on joint inflammation in both lab animals and humans. Many people have gotten dramatic relief from taking these out of their diet completely. A very good article on this appeared in the *Journal of Neurological and Orthopedic Medical Surgery* (v. 12, 1993), containing a long list of references. Solanine poisoning has various effects we still do not know about. The known ones include nausea, diarrhea, abdominal cramps, coma, fever, headache, weak pulse, delirium, rapid breathing, and hallucinations. We need more research here, especially on humans. There have been recorded incidents of mass poisoning in Europe earlier in the last century, when poor people ate large amounts of potatoes, as they had no other food to eat.

THE MACROBIOTIC NATURAL ORDER

Macrobiotic philosophy was really the only system of eating to tell people in temperate climates not to eat tropical foods. Other diets seem to ignore this very obvious fact. Foods grown in tropical areas are extremely yin, to balance their extremely yang environment. Nature has a pattern here. The foods that grow in hot tropical climates, like mangoes, bananas, papayas, citrus fruit, avocados, taro, and coconuts, are meant for the indigenous peoples in those areas, helping them to adapt to such a climate. Modern transportation makes tropical foods easily and inexpensively available all year round now.

Nature gives us the foods we need, in the native climate we live in. If you fed an Inuit such tropical foods they would sicken and die quickly. On the other hand, if you fed someone in Southern India nothing but fish, seal meat, and whale fat, they would also sicken and die quickly. The situation gets much more confusing when people of European descent move to tropical areas to live. The same situation exists when people from Africa, the Philippines, or Southern India move to temperate climates to make their home. All these people are going against the order of the universe, and not harmonizing their genetics with their environment. Take people of African descent, for example. In Africa there really is very little typical western disease, such as various cancers—breast, ovarian, uterine, cervical, lung, and prostate, diabetes, high blood pressure, atherosclerosis, and heart attacks. Men and women of African descent who live in America and Europe have stratospheric rates of all these diseases, from an environment and diet not meant for their genetics. The same is true for Europeans who move to tropical climates. This is what happens when you are out of tune with the universal order. *Our bodies are a microcosm of the universe,* and we also are microcosms of the environment we live in. Stay in harmony with the Natural Order.

Have you ever noticed that vitamin C is basically only found in any quantity in tropical fruits (also in the nightshade fruit tomatoes) like mangos, papayas, citrus fruits, and the like? These fruits are meant for the indigenous peoples of hot tropical areas. They need more vitamin C than we do. There is sufficient vitamin C in the fresh green and yellow vegetables we eat in temperate climates. We have no need at all to eat tropical fruits, or take vitamin C supplements. In fact, this is clearly counterproductive. This very yin vitamin (ascorbic acid) acidifies our normally alkaline blood. The United States in recent years has a very high consumption of various citrus fruits and citrus juice, for example. Orange juice for breakfast is an American tradition. Citrus fruits are plentiful, inexpensive, and widely consumed, and contribute very much to the bad health of our country. This is especially true when these very acidic fruits, high in vitamin C, are eaten in the winter time, which is very yin. Since citrus fruit is very inexpensive and available year round, this has become a staple in American culture. When people have a cold or flu, they are often told to drink more orange and grapefruit juice! This just makes them worse, of course. You find most all vegetarians are sugar addicts, and eat large amounts of sweet tropical fruits such as mangoes and bananas, natural sweeteners such as honey, dried fruit, and fruit juice. They think these are good for them. Sugar is sugar is sugar, and all simple mono- and disaccharides have the same basic deleterious effects when eaten in any quantity.

Avocados are a popular fruit because of their very high (78 percent) fat content. One cup of Hass avocado contains a whopping 407 calories, four-fifths of which are from fat—36 grams of fat. Avocados are almost 80 percent fat calories! Most vegetarians eat many tropical fruits such as avocados regularly. One more reason vegetarianism, as practiced, does not work very well. There is no understanding of the Order of the Universe here.

CONCLUSION

The point is for genetically temperate people to eat foods that grow in colder climates, and avoid foods that grow in tropical climates. In his book *Man, the Unknown,* Alexis Carrel writes, "Man is literally made from the dust of the earth. For this reason, his physiological and mental activities are profoundly influenced by the geological constitution of the country where he lives, by the nature of the animals and plants he eats." We are healthier, stronger, and in tune with the universal laws when we eat the food in our environment that was given to us by Nature to be appropriate.

7. Fruits and Sugars

People are usually very surprised to find that eating fruit is generally limited in macrobiotics, except in small amounts, and only locally grown fruits. One serving a day of fresh fruit is enough. People with blood sugar problems should eat no fruit, fruit juice, or sweeteners whatsoever until they are well. If you look at a nutrition profile of almost any fruit, you will find it is basically just water, sugar, a little fiber, and almost no vitamins, minerals, or other nutrients. Fruits are simply a poor source of nutrition, and contain large amounts of simple sugars, especially sucrose and fructose. That's right, the same white sugar (sucrose) and the same fructose (as high-fructose corn syrup) you find in junk foods. *Sugar is sugar is sugar.*

Almost all vegetarians, especially vegans, are addicted to simple sugars. They eat far too much honey, dried fruits, raw sugar, fruit juices, maple syrup, tropical fruits, stevia, agave syrup, desserts, and other sweets. They rationalize this by saying these are natural sugars. Again, all sugars are natural. There is no reason at all to eat desserts at the end of a meal. You'll be better off if you take the concept of dessert out of your dietary regimen. At first, you may be attached to sweets. Get a macrobiotic dessert cookbook like Meredith McCarty's *Sweet and Natural*, and learn how to make desserts out of whole grains and unsweetened fruit. Remember, this is a temporary stage, and not something to continue. Have you noticed that most all Asian cultures do not embrace the idea of desserts at the end of the meal? This is a very good practice to adopt in your own life. *You don't need desserts.* Begin your meal with soup instead.

NUTRITIONAL VALUE

We are constantly told to eat more fresh fruits, but fruits have very little nutrition. This is proven by laboratory analysis. There are almost no minerals in fruit. We are known to need at least twenty minerals, and you just won't get these from fruits. The situation is hardly any better with the thirteen vitamins we need, even though a few fruits do contain some vitamin A, beta carotene, and vitamin C. Definitely fruit juice, fruit concentrate, and dried fruits should be avoided, as these are concentrated sugars. Remember that all sugar is sugar, and all sugar is natural. Whether you use white sugar, brown sugar, raw sugar, molasses, honey, maple syrup, date sugar, fructose, corn syrup, agave, xylitol, cane sugar, maltose, or amazake, you are still eating simple sugars. Stevia has the same negative effects on your health, and sucralose is a chemical abomination. Basically, they are all the same in biological effect. You need no fruit in your diet at all, actually, and the only practical reason to eat it is for variety and taste. *Fruit is very low in all known nutrients.*

Fruits generally contain very, very little mineral content such as calcium, magnesium, iron, copper, iodine, zinc, manganese, selenium, boron, vanadium, strontium, nickel, tin, molybdenum, germanium, chromium, silicon, cesium, gallium, rubidium, and cobalt. Let's take twelve of the most commonly eaten, representative fruits, and see how many minerals are in them —apples, apricots, bananas, blueberries, cantaloupe, grapes, oranges, peaches, pears, pineapples, plums, and strawberries. You would have to eat:

- **Calcium**—about 12 pounds of these common fruits to get even 400 mg.

- **Copper**—10 pounds to get 2 mg.

- **Iron**—15 pounds of fruit to get 15 mg.

- **Magnesium**—about 8 pounds to get just 250 mg.

- **Manganese**—4 pounds to get 2 mg.

- **Selenium** or **Chromium**—there is virtually none in fruit.

- **Zinc**—40 pounds to get 15 mg.

You can see that fruit is not going to significantly contribute any of these vital elements to your diet.

There are only thirteen vitamins, and while some fruits do in fact contain some vitamin A (or beta carotene) or vitamin C, they are a very poor source of all the others. Fruit contains no vitamin D, and very little E, K, thiamine, riboflavin, niacin, B_6, B_{12}, pantothenic acid, folic acid, or biotin. Let's take the same group of twelve common fruits above, and see how much vitamin content they have

- **Vitamin A** (or beta carotene)—the Recommended Dietary Allowance is 5,000 International Units (IU). There is no RDA for beta carotene, but a healthy dose is 10,000 IU. A few fruits, such as cantaloupe or apricots, contain good amounts of vitamin A or beta carotene (the direct precursor). Most fruits, such as apples and pears, contain almost none. You would need to eat almost a hundred pounds of apples or pears to get what you need! Fruit generally is not even a good source of vitamin A or beta carotene.

- **Vitamin B_1** (thiamine)—the RDA is 1.5 mg. There is almost no thiamine in any fruits. You would have to eat over ten pounds of mixed apples, bananas, pears, oranges, and strawberries to get what you need.

- **Vitamin B_2** (riboflavin)—the RDA is 1.7 mg. There is almost no riboflavin in any fruits. You would need to eat over twelve pounds of mixed apples, bananas, pears, oranges, and strawberries to get what you need.

- **Vitamin B_3** (niacin)—the RDA is 20 mg. There is almost no niacin in any fruits. You would have to eat about thirty pounds of mixed apples, bananas, pears, oranges (one of the best sources), and strawberries to get what you need.

- **Vitamin B_5** (pantothenic acid)—the RDA is 10 mg. Again, most fruits have almost no pantothenic acid, with few exceptions. Strawberries are one of the best sources, yet you would have to eat ten pounds to get a mere 10 mg.

- **Vitamin B_6**—the RDA is 2 mg. There is very little B_6 in most fruits. You would have to eat about ten pounds of mixed apples, bananas, pears, oranges, and strawberries to get what you need.

- **Vitamin B_7 (biotin)**—the RDA is 300 mcg. There is just not enough biotin in any fruit to mention. You would have to eat fifty pounds of oranges to get what you need, and that is one of the best sources.

- **Vitamin B_9 (folic acid)**—the RDA is 400 mcg. Folate is found in small quantities in a few fruits. You would still have to eat about three pounds of common fruit to get what you need. You would literally have to eat over eighty pounds of apples, however.

- **Vitamin B_{12}**—the RDA is a mere 2.4 mcg. Basically, there is just no vitamin B_{12} in fruits. We synthesize the B_{12} we need in our intestines. (Make sure your vitamin supplement contains methyl cobalamin, and not regular B_{12}, as it just won't be absorbed.)

• **Vitamin C**—the RDA is 60 mg. You'll notice that basically only tropical fruits, such as citrus and mangoes, contain any appreciable amount of vitamin C. Temperate fruits, such as apples, grapes, and peaches, contain very little vitamin C. You would have to eat about eight pounds of these to get the 60 mg you need. Tropical people in tropical climates, need higher levels of vitamin C, and nature has provided this. Temperate people in temperate climates, are meant by Nature to consume much less of this very yin vitamin.

• **Vitamin D**—the RDA is 400 IU. There is no Vitamin D in any plant food; no fruit contains any vitamin D. Vitamin D is, in fact, a hormone, and not a vitamin at all. It is found in very small amounts in some animal foods such as eggs. You can only get sufficient amounts by exposure to the sun, or taking vitamin D_3 supplements. Take only 400 to 1,200 IU if you are not in the sun regularly. Do not exceed this amount. This is fat soluble and accumulates in the body.

• **Vitamin E**—the RDA is 30 IU. Fruits are remarkably deficient in vitamin E. Apples and peaches are some of the best sources, yet you would have to eat about ten pounds of either to get what you need. Your best source of vitamin E is whole grains.

• **Vitamin K**—the RDA is 80 micrograms (mcg). Fruit is also remarkably deficient in vitamin K. There are very few exceptions, such as peaches (8 mcg per 100 g serving). Some fruits have none at all.

Fruits are a very optional part of your diet. They are good for variety, and to make our food more appealing.

CHOOSING YOUR FRUITS

If you choose to include fruit in your diet, pick temperate ones like plums, berries, peaches, cherries, apples, grapes, and such. Do not eat tropical fruits like coconuts, guavas, mangoes, papayas, bananas, avocadoes, and others. These are meant for tropical races living in their native climates. If you are of, say, South American, African or Indian ancestry, and living in a hot climate where these foods are grown, then you certainly can enjoy them on a daily basis. This is discussed in Chapter 6. The best time of year to include one serving of fruit a day in your diet is summer time, when nature makes it available. Fruits are very yin, and more appropriate in the yang summer time. The least desirable time is in the winter, when they are not naturally available. People of temperate genetics living in hot, yang, sunny areas like southern Florida or southern California should not rationalize this as a reason to eat tropical fruit.

EFFECTS OF SUGAR INTAKE

Diabetes, metabolic syndrome, hyperglycemia, hypoglycemia, insulin resistance, and other blood sugar disorders are epidemic. One big reason is the inordinate intake of about 160 pounds of various sugars per year in our diets. Most of this comes from high-fructose corn syrup, since it is the cheapest to manufacture. Imagine scarfing down more than three pounds of different sugars every week! Refined grains, excessive fat intake, obesity, and lack of exercise are other reasons for blood sugar problems. Whole grains slowly metabolized into blood glucose, which is used as needed. Doctors are still irrationally recommending harmful high-protein diets for such people. These patients then end up on toxic, ineffective prescription drugs for the rest of their lives. When you eat a high-protein diet, you have to eat a lot of saturated fat and cholesterol as well. Adult onset diabetes, along with insulin resistance, are the biggest health epidemics in the world now. (Insulin resistance means the body produces enough insulin, but the cells don't metabolize it well.) Your fasting blood sugar should be 85 mg or less. The medical goal of 100 mg or less is just not valid. If it is higher than 85 mg, get an inexpensive one-draw glucose tolerance test (GTT). Some people have normal blood sugar levels, yet still suffer from insulin resistance. The HbA1c test is another tool. A minority, on the other hand, suffer from low blood sugar, or hypoglycemia. The symptoms here are constant hunger—even after eating—weakness and fatigue, perspiring too much, yawning inappropriately, and emotional swings.

CONCLUSION

Macrobiotic diets generally limit fruit consumption to seasonal and locally grown fruits, and to at most one serving a day. Remember, if you live in a temperate climate, bypass tropical fruits, and feed on only temperate climate fruits. As we have seen in this chapter, there are certain health dangers that are associated with the habitual consumption of sugar and sugar products, which are devoid of any nutritional value.

8. Seafood, Meat, Poultry, and Dairy

You can choose to be a vegetarian for health, for ethical reasons, or both. People on a meditative spiritual path will often choose not to eat any type of animal food. You can eat a purely plant-based diet if you want. You will find that vegans and ethical vegetarians are usually not really health oriented. They always eat an inordinate amount of various sugars. The macrobiotic diet can include most any type of seafood in moderation, especially during the winter, and in cold climates. Moderation would mean a small four-to six-ounce portion, say, five times a week. It is best to eat lower-calorie, lower-fat white-fleshed fish like cod, perch, flounder, grouper, sole, halibut, haddock, and other varieties. Shellfish such as crab, shrimp, scallops, clams, oysters, and lobster are also good choices. It is best to minimize, or avoid, the high-fat white fish like catfish, orange roughy, and turbot. The same applies to red-fleshed fish like tuna, mackerel, salmon, and swordfish. It is a biological and physiological fact that our teeth and digestive systems are designed to eat small amounts of animal food. Seafood is the healthiest animal food to eat. You can see from the chart on page 39 that the fat content of seafood varies dramatically from 7 percent to 52 percent. A three and a third ounce (100 g) portion of seafood generally is low in fat, has less than 100 calories, and is very filling on a caloric basis.

DAIRY

Dairy products are also eaten by some people who call themselves vegetarians. This is irrational, since milk is not a plant-based food. Whether the milk and dairy products are organically produced is beside the point, and does not change the basic nature of them. What is wrong with dairy products? They contain lactose and casein. *Milk is the number one worst allergen of all known foods.* No other food is a universal allergen like milk and the products derived from milk. Whole milk is an amazing 48 percent fat calories. To learn more about the many reasons not to drink milk or eat dairy products, go to websites such as www.notmilk.com and read what they have to say. Cow milk is meant for calves, not human babies, and certainly not human adults. The lactose and casein are deleterious. *All adults of all races are lactose intolerant.* That's a scientific fact. Every biologist knows that all mammals lose the ability to produce the enzyme lactase soon after birth and weaning. Lactose (milk sugar) does not just pass through your digestive system like fiber, but causes allergic reactions. Casein is a proven carcinogen.

There are a lot of other reasons not to eat dairy products, even if you go to the trouble and expense of buying organic and low-fat varieties. There are now tasty, inexpensive, and readily available soy, rice, oat, flax, and almond nondairy alternatives to most dairy products. You can find nondairy sour cream, yogurt, many flavors of meltable cheese, and cream cheese. There is just no reason to eat dairy products. Yogurt has long been considered a health food by most people, but is certainly not healthy. Yogurt contains twice the lactose of regular milk, because milk powder is added to thicken it. The soy yogurts currently available are certainly tasty, but have too much sugar in them. Hard cheeses contain little lactose, but are so full of saturated fat and cholesterol as to make it a poor food choice. Soy cheese comes in at least ten flavors now, melts easily, tastes similar to dairy cheese, but is rich in vegetable oil and should be used in moderation. Soy ice cream has as much sugar as regular ice cream. Dairy sour cream, cream, cream cheese and all the rest are very unhealthy foods to eat. The least objectionable dairy food is low-fat cottage cheese. While low-fat cottage cheese has very little lactose and fat, it contains a lot of cancer promoting casein.

MEAT

Americans eat twice the protein they need. There is just no reason to eat red meat such as beef, pork, lamb, or wild meats such as venison, rabbit, and squirrel. Excess protein promotes cancer, and causes such problems as high uric acid and kidney disease. Excess protein also creates an unbalanced bacterial environment in our intestines. Animal proteins are very different from vegetable proteins. Like animal fats, they are highly correlated with many diseases, including kidney disease, diabetes, arthritis, coronary heart disease (CHD), and cancers of various types. *High-protein diets are actually harm-*

ful to your health. Protein is not a good energy source, as it must be broken down in steps, which leave toxic byproducts in our blood. Whole grains, on the other hand, are an excellent direct energy source, and do not leave unwanted byproducts as they are digested. We only need about 0.6 grams of protein per kilogram of body weight. A 150-pound person only needs about 40 grams of protein every day. The high-protein crowd advises eating a gram of protein for every pound of body weight (150 grams per 150 pound person), which is very unhealthy. You get all the protein you need by eating a variety of whole grains, beans, and vegetables. *We do not need animal foods as a source of protein.*

Regarding red meat, there are two reasons not to eat cows, pigs, sheep, deer, chickens, turkeys, and other animals. In Buddhism, "ahimsa," or doing no harm, is a basic tenet. *We do not need to kill animals to eat.* We do this only for sensory pleasure. If you are going to eat meat or poultry, then be honest with yourself about the life you are taking. If you had to personally kill and butcher a cow, chicken, pig, or turkey, or especially a calf or a young lamb, would you still be eating them? If you were directly responsible for their deaths, how much meat and poultry would you really be eating? The second reason is biological. We are biologically equipped to basically eat plant foods due to our digestive systems and our teeth.

POULTRY

Poultry and eggs, organic or not, are two of the top ten allergenic foods known, and these should be avoided. Taking these out of your diet in our culture can be very difficult, because they are inexpensive, found almost everywhere, and served in a wide variety of ways. Some people eat eggs, yet call themselves vegetarians. It makes no difference whether an egg is organically produced, fertile, free range, or anything else. *They are still eggs,* and should not be eaten. *Whole eggs are 50 percent fat calories, and contain a whopping 250 mg of cholesterol.* Some people just eat the egg whites, but they are just as allergenic as the yolks and are still animal proteins. Poultry, even when steamed or broiled without the skin, is neither a healthy food nor even a low-fat food. It is full of fat and cholesterol.

SEAFOOD

Seafood is the best choice of protein if you choose not to be a vegetarian. Seafood is better suited for men rather than women, for hard-working people, those who are physically active and exercise a lot, in the colder seasons (it is very yang), and for people who live in cold climates. Seafood should be limited in warmer climates and in the summertime. A small percent of people have a generalized allergy to fish and/or shellfish. Such allergies should be obvious if they exist, but some allergies are more hidden and subtle. It is best to choose shellfish and light-fleshed, low-fat fish such as cod, flounder, sole, and others, over dark-fleshed, high-fat fish such as tuna, swordfish, and salmon.

TABLE 8.1. CALORIES AND FAT CALORIES IN COMMON SEAFOOD 100 GRAM PORTIONS (RAW)

Fish	cal.	fat cal.	Fish	cal.	fat cal.
Catfish	110	33	Halibut	103	19
Turbot	90	28	Flounder	84	7
Perch	89	11	Snapper	94	11
Cod	79	7	King Crab	78	13
Swordfish	114	26	Blue Crab	82	11
Salmon	135	31	Clams	70	11
Mackerel	131	38	Mussels	81	23
Scallops	83	7	Mahi	80	7
Seatrout	97	31	Grouper	86	10
Lobster	106	10	Oysters	76	25
Sole	64	8	Ocean Perch	94	11
Tuna	135	30	Squid	86	12
Rockfish	89	11	Shrimp	100	10
Kingfish	100	26	Carp	119	40
Haddock	110	7	Herring	149	52
Monkfish	71	14	Pollack	86	10
Sea Bass	90	19	Orange Roughy	119	49
Shark	123	31	Croaker	99	27

SCIENTIFIC STUDIES

A study was done at the University of Manchester in England on milk intake and death from coronary heart disease (CHD)—the largest killer of all of both men and women. The populations of forty different countries were studied. You can see the death rate is much lower in populations who drink very little or no milk. The men who drank the most milk had the highest death rate. Finland had literally one thousand men per hundred thousand die from heart disease every single year, yet they drank only one cup of milk per 1,000 calories of food intake. This chart is based on millions of men in forty different countries and simply cannot be disputed. *Milk is very bad food.*

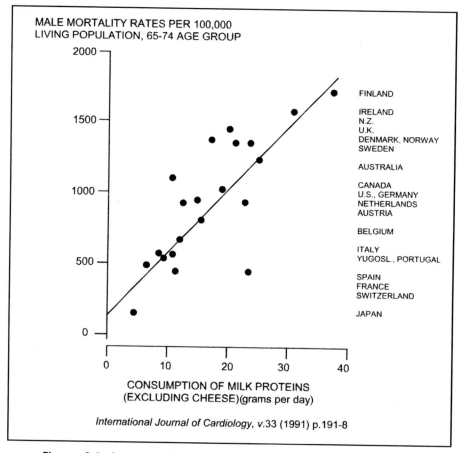

MALE MORTALITY RATES PER 100,000 LIVING POPULATION, 65-74 AGE GROUP

FINLAND

IRELAND
N.Z.
U.K.
DENMARK, NORWAY
SWEDEN

AUSTRALIA

CANADA
U.S., GERMANY
NETHERLANDS
AUSTRIA

BELGIUM

ITALY
YUGOSL., PORTUGAL

SPAIN
FRANCE
SWITZERLAND

JAPAN

CONSUMPTION OF MILK PROTEINS
(EXCLUDING CHEESE)(grams per day)

International Journal of Cardiology, v.33 (1991) p.191-8

Figure 8.1. Consumption of Milk Proteins (Excluding Cheese)
The chart above illustrates that the more milk you drink, the shorter your life expectancy.

Milk and dairy products are full of lactose, casein, pesticides, herbicides, bacteria, viruses, antibiotics, hormones, and dioxins. Milk is simply liquid meat due to the animal proteins, especially casein. Casein is very allergenic and only found in milk. Three glasses of milk contain more cholesterol than a dozen strips of bacon. Yogurt is two times more cholesterol-concentrated, cheese is ten times more cholesterol-concentrated, ice cream is twelve times concentrated, and butter is an amazing twenty-one times concentrated—99 percent fat calories. Drinking milk and eating dairy products have been linked to obesity, coronary heart disease, various cancers and malignancies, liver disease, diabetes and blood sugar disorders, kidney disease, multiple sclerosis, and Crohn's disease, among many other illnesses.

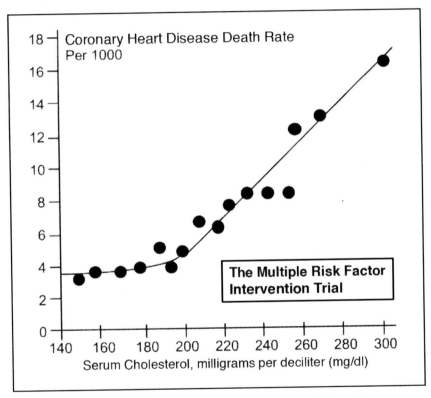

Figure 8.2. High Cholesterol Means High Mortality

This Multiple Risk Factor Intervention Trial was one of the largest and longest of all human studies on heart and artery health. This chart above is based on 361,662 people, thirty-five to fifty-seven years old, studied over a period of six years. You can see that people who eat a low-fat diet and have a cholesterol level of about 150 mg/dl have the fewest deaths of all from heart and artery disease. The average American has a cholesterol level of about 250 mg/dl, and suffers about 250 percent greater risk of death every year than citizens of other countries. The medical profession tells you that a total cholesterol level of 200 mg/dl or less is the ideal. *The real goal is about 150 mg/dl.* This is the level you'll generally find in rural Asians as a group. Their coronary heart disease (CHD) rates are a fraction of ours. *The lower your cholesterol is, the better.* The only food source of cholesterol is animal products such as meat, poultry, eggs, and dairy products. Seafood in moderation does not raise your cholesterol level. There is no cholesterol in any plant food.

The Framingham Study was the largest human study ever done, and came to the very same conclusions. People who tell you cholesterol doesn't count are just making excuses for eating red meat and other high-fat foods. *Total cholesterol is the single best indicator of heart and artery health, and of longevity.*

CONCLUSION

There is no doubt that eating meat, dairy, poultry, and eggs result in far more disease of every kind, less quality of life, and a shorter lifespan. The longest lived people on earth are the Okinawans. Their basic diet is grains, root vegetables, leafy vegetables, and seafood. They eat very small amounts of animal foods such as pork, chicken, and eggs. You can't argue with real-world proof like this. Read T. Colin Campbell and Thomas M. Campbell's book *The China Study* for more on this.

9. Fats and Oils

It is important that you eat a low-fat diet for many reasons. There are only three sources of calories—carbohydrates at 5 calories per gram, proteins at 5 calories, and fats at 9 calories per gram. Fats of all kinds contain almost twice the calories of carbohydrates or proteins. Since you will not be eating red meat, poultry, eggs, milk, or dairy products, it is really quite easy to keep your fat calorie intake down to 10 or 15 percent. *Twenty percent is the very maximum* and there is no reason to eat that much. Do not think that vegetable oils are somehow good for you, as unsaturated vegetable oils are less harmful than saturated animal fats. Clinical studies have shown that vegetable oils can sometimes promote cancer cell growth as well as the saturated fats. Saturated fats are basically only found in animal foods. Palm and coconut are the most saturated plant oils, and are meant for tropical people in hot climates. The fats in fish and seafood are not harmful in moderation, and do not raise your cholesterol and triglyceride levels.

OILS

You actually do not need any vegetable oils in your kitchen, and many people simply do not use these in their food preparation. You can use oils in moderation for stir-frying, baking, salad dressing, and other limited uses. Which oils are good for general use? All the oils you see in the grocery store are generally heavily refined, heated to high temperatures, and filtered to make them clear and more visually appealing.

● **Extra-virgin olive oil** is about the only exception. The cold-pressed oils in the natural food store are quite pricey. You are getting very little nutrition from oil anyway, and you will be using very little of them, so cold-pressed oils are not necessary. Also, any solvents that are used to extract oil are boiled off completely.

- **Corn oil** is a fine choice, especially since it comes from grain.

- **Safflower and sunflower oils**, both polyunsaturated oils, are good choices.

- **Sesame oil** is good, but just too expensive for general use.

- **Toasted sesame or dark sesame oil** is an excellent condiment for Asian dishes.

- **Olive oil** is a good choice, but it is no better than other vegetable oils.

- **Soy oil** does not taste good unless it has been very heavily refined.

- **Peanut oil** comes from one of the top ten allergenic foods, and is not a good choice at all.

- **Cottonseed oil** is purely a commercial byproduct of the cotton industry, and was never meant for human consumption. It is a favorite oil for hydrogenation since it is the least expensive edible oil. Avoid anything that has the generic description "vegetable oil" or "vegetable oil blend." You can bet this is a cheap cottonseed oil.

- **Walnut, avocado, pumpkin seed, almond, grape seed, and other gourmet oils** make nice specialty oils, but are very expensive and have limited use.

- **Palm and coconut oils** are tropical foods, and should only be used occasionally. Coconut oil is not a health supplement.

   Canola oil needs a separate mention. The made-up name comes from "Canadian oil," and is from the rapeseed (from the Latin "rapa" or turnip) plant. This is promoted in the natural foods industry as a healthy oil to use, when it certainly is not. Canola oil, by law, must contain less than 2 percent of the toxic erucic acid that is naturally contained in it. For many years rapeseed oil could only be fed to farm animals, or used in industrial applications because of the high erucic acid content. This is a major crop in the cold Canadian climate. The farmers genetically engineered this, over the years, to make it acceptable for human use. *This was never meant for human consumption,* and no amount of genetic engineering will make it so. Do not buy or use products with canola oil, no matter how promoted they are in the so-called natural foods industry. The real motivation here is profit. *Do not use canola oil.*

FATS

Americans eat more fat than anyone on earth. On the average, people in America eat an astounding 42 percent fat calories, and most of these are from animal fats. Five times the amount of fats we need, and the wrong kind of fats! Plus, we consume twice the protein, twice the calories, refined foods, preservatives, and 160 pounds of various sugars. Then we wonder why we have the highest disease rates in the world!

Rural Asians and macrobiotic dieters have cholesterol levels of about 150 mg/dl, triglyceride levels under 100 mg/dl, and excellent HDL to LDL ratios. Total cholesterol is an excellent predictor of life span. Such people also have very low cancer rates, as you can see by the following charts on breast and prostate cancer. Men with very low fat intake, especially animal fats, rarely get prostate disease of any kind. Women who do the same rarely get breast, ovarian, cervical, uterine, or other cancers.

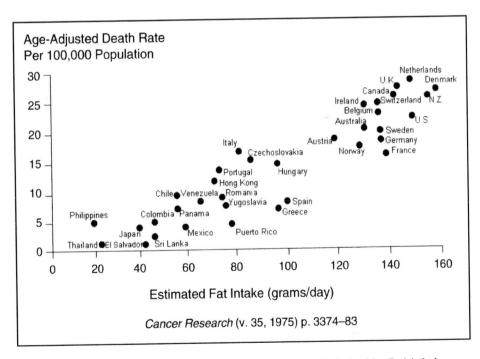

Figure 9.1. International Breast Cancer Rates Related to Fat Intake

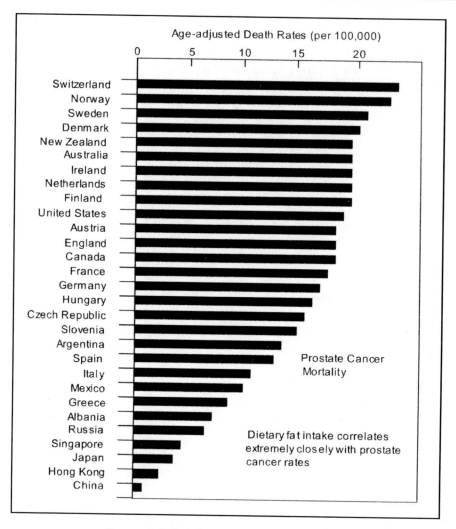

Figure 9.2. Fat Causes Prostate Cancer

CONCLUSION

An American's diet consists of more than 40 percent saturated animal fats. You should eat less than 20 percent vegetable oils and preferably no more than 15 percent. Excess dietary fat of any kind is harmful. You need to keep your total cholesterol down to 150 mg/dl and your triglycerides under 100 mg/dl. Corn, safflower, sunflower, and olive oils are good everyday choices. It is easy to eat a low-fat diet of whole grains, beans, vegetables, fruits, soups, salads, and seafood.

10. Condiments and Seasonings

Eating should be fun, delicious, and most enjoyable. One of the reasons Japanese macrobiotics is understandably not appealing to many people is the severe and very unnecessary restrictions on seasonings and condiments. Eating this way is just not very tasty, fun, or enjoyable. The flavors seem to be limited to such things as tamari soy sauce, ginger root, miso, bonito shavings, natto, sesame seeds, and few other Japanese traditions. *There is just no good reason for this.* Food should be delicious, flavorful, aesthetic, pleasing, and fully seasoned without the use of fats and hot spices.

USING CONDIMENTS AND SEASONINGS IN FOOD

The key to using the following seasonings is *moderation.* There are many flavorings that can enhance your food when used with a light hand. Herbs such as sage, rosemary, basil, thyme, tarragon, oregano, bay leaf, cumin, marjoram, mint, lemongrass, caraway seed, celery seed, good vinegars, horseradish, Italian seasoning, mustard, nutmeg, garlic, coriander leaf and seed, parsley, orange peel, lemon and lime peel, lemon and lime juice (in small amounts), Chinese soy sauce, dry sherry, vanilla, Thai fish sauce, Old Bay seasoning, Worcestershire sauce, and capers are all good. It is true we should avoid, or limit, powerful hot spices such as black pepper, cayenne pepper, chilies, hot sauce, and other such strong condiments.

47

SOY PRODUCTS

Soybean-based products may be used as a flavor enhancer or as garnish. Miso is a salty, fermented seasoning paste and it may also be used as a thickener. Soy sauce, also made from fermented soybeans, is very often used as a condiment or as a seasoning in cooking. Soy cheese in a variety of flavors, soy milk, soy yogurt, soy sour cream, and other soy products will replace most dairy products.

NUTS

Toasted nuts such as walnuts, almonds, pine nuts, filberts, and pecans make an elegant garnish, especially to stir-fried vegetables. *Nuts are a garnish and not a food per se.* Limit the use of nut butters such as almond or soy nut butter, as the fat content is far too high. Nuts are only a garnish to enhance our meals.

SALT

The most important condiment to talk about is salt. The word salt comes from the Latin word "sal." Salt is what the word "salary" is based on, since Roman soldiers were paid in part with salt. Salt was one of the most important items of commerce for thousands of years, and still is. The Bible is full of references to salt. We've all heard the term, "salt of the earth." We need salt in our diet, although some people will tell you not to use any salt at all. The Framingham Study proved, beyond any doubt, that moderate salt use is not harmful and does not contribute to high blood pressure or any other coronary heart condition. Americans overall do eat too much salt and sodium from processed foods and over-salting their meals. No unprocessed food contains a lot of sodium. Salt in moderation is necessary in our diet, and should be used reasonably in our food. Salt-free diets are dull, boring, very unnecessary, and unhealthful in the long term.

Traditional macrobiotics simply used too much salt in such things as miso, miso soup, tamari soy sauce, natto, gomasio (ground sesame seeds and salt), pickled vegetables, and pressed salads. You do not need to buy overpriced "sea salt," as all salt comes from the sea. That's right—all salt originated in the oceans, and has been deposited on land. The tiny amounts of minerals this provides are biologically insignificant, consisting mostly of very small amounts of magnesium. Simply find a brand of salt that does not use an aluminum anti-caking agent (always avoid anything with aluminum salts in it). Our bodies naturally expel salt in the urine within hours of taking it in, but that is no reason to overdo it. Eating too much salt results in edema (water retention), unbalances the body, and uses up valuable energy getting rid of the excess water. Use salt intelligently in moderation.

BAKING POWDER

Baking powder and baking soda are not used in macrobiotics, and this is very smart. If you want to bake something occasionally that cannot be leavened with yeast, find a sodium-based baking powder like Rumford. Do not eat such things as baking powder biscuits with any regularity, as both baking powder and baking soda are extremely yin. Never eat anything with aluminum based baking powder, as this is one of the main sources of aluminum in our diets. Aluminum pots are rarely used anymore. Aluminum cookware is now almost always coated with chemically inert Teflon. There is no reason not to use Teflon cookware either. It is chemically inert, even at normal cooking temperatures. You can use aluminum foil except with acidic foods. Use stainless steel pans for really hot stir frying. Aluminum-based underarm deodorants are transdermal, and a very major source of aluminum in our systems, by the way. Nearly all commercial deodorants use aluminum salts.

CONDIMENTS TO AVOID

Avoid peanut butter, as it is too allergenic. Avoid tomato-based condiments such as ketchup and barbeque sauce. Mayonnaise is obviously too full of fat for regular use. Most salad dressings are full of fats and chemicals. Make your own light salad dressings.

CONCLUSION

Cooking is a joyous art. Seasonings should generally be added during the preparation of food. Condiments can be made available at the table to allow for one to individually adjust taste, and garnishes may be added to make the meal more appealing. Flavor your foods well, without fat, and enjoy them.

11. Everyday Eating

Eat two meals a day. Eating two meals a day just makes life simpler and makes you healthier. Thoreau said, "Simplify, simplify, simplify." Eating two meals a day makes it far easier to cook, to eat well, to make good food choices, to limit your caloric intake while not being hungry, and to not eat out as much. Ideally, choose a small breakfast or lunch, and eat a main evening meal. This two-meal-a-day plan allows you to have a healthier digestive system. This is the best way to live, but it can take a while to achieve this and not be hungry. Men only need about 1,800 calories a day and women only about 1,200 calories. You're not going to reach that goal with three meals.

MAKING MEALS ENJOYABLE

This way of eating and drinking *should be fun,* and not dull, boring, bland, or restrictive. When you see the very wide range of healthy, delicious, whole natural grains, beans, green and yellow vegetables, seafood, salads, and local fruits that are included, you do not feel limited at all. You can modify many Asian, Northern Italian, country French, Mexican, Latin, Mediterranean, Middle Eastern, and South American recipes so they are in tune with universal principles.

● Indian food uses too much dairy and tropical condiments such as fenugreek, pepper, cumin, hot chilies, mustard, coconut milk, cardamon, tamarind, cayenne, and other yin-stimulating spices for regular use. Burmese, Cambodian, Tibetan, and Filipino foods are exotic, different, and interesting.

- Southern Italian cooking uses red meat, poultry, eggs, white pasta, white bread, dairy products, endless tomatoes, and lots of cheese. It is very hard to substitute for tomatoes in cooking, due to their unique flavor.

- The much-promoted Mediterranean diet just does not cut it. This diet includes white bread, white pasta, cheese, tomatoes, and far too much olive oil.

- Northern Italian cooking uses too much meat and cheese.

- Thai cooking uses too many tropical spices like hot chilies, curries (different from Indian curry), peppers, and coconut milk for regular use.

- Vietnamese cooking offers many possibilities with only small changes.

- Korean cooking has potential, but is the least healthy of all Asian cooking styles.

- Cajun cooking has little to offer, due to its highly spicy nature and use of animal foods and fats.

- Eastern European cooking uses meat, poultry, potatoes, dairy products, and refined grains.

- Classical Northern European (English, Welsh, Irish, Scottish, German, Swiss, and Austrian) cooking is a meat-and-potatoes diet by tradition.

- French country cooking is definitely better than the high-fat classic French, and has some good potential if used creatively.

- Central and South American cooking offer possibilities when whole grains are used and tropical fruits and nightshade vegetables are omitted.

- Middle Eastern food can be very applicable to whole-grain healthy meals.

- Mexican cooking has possibilities due to the beans, rice, and tortillas, when you take the cheese and meat out of it. They use very little green and yellow vegetables, however.

- Soul food uses too many animal products and deep frying.

- Generally, the healthiest recipes are going to come from the Asian countries. Most people find the various regional Chinese styles to be the most practical and enjoyable, especially the stir-fried vegetables.

- There is a lot you can do with standard American cooking, and some imagination to make healthful meals.

Get some cookbooks from your local library for new and creative ideas. Learn how to cook and season the foods you already eat in new and better ways. See the Recommended Reading on page 107.

FOODS TO EAT

Since you will only be eating two meals a day, life is going to be much simpler. Would you rather drop breakfast or drop lunch? Or you can vary this day to day depending on your mood. Since working people often have so little time, and are so hurried in the morning, it might be better to eat only lunch and dinner. If you do prefer to eat breakfast, make it light, with hot or cold whole grain cereal, whole grain bread, nondairy milk, and herbal tea. Soy milk contains about 120 calories per cup, so this isn't good as a daily beverage (this would add over 800 calories a week). The American tradition of orange juice for breakfast is not a good one. Regular tea is full of caffeine, and coffee is not part of a healthy lifestyle.

It is a good idea to take your own lunch to work every day for a lot of reasons. A good lunch would include brown rice or other grain, a green or yellow vegetable, a thermos of hot soup, beans, fresh salad, and good bread. You can learn to make very interesting sandwiches without meat, poultry or dairy. Most offices have facilities for people who bring their lunch. You can eat a much more delicious meal from home than eating in a restaurant.

Dinner should be the main meal of the day. A whole grain should be your principal food, of course. A good dinner would not be very different from lunch. A whole grain or whole wheat pasta, beans, a green or yellow vegetable, some seafood if desired, and bread, soup, or salad. The idea of dessert is mostly a western one. You can temporarily fix macrobiotic desserts, but only as a transition. Enjoy a piece of local fruit, especially in warm climates, and in summer, if you feel the need for something sweet. You will be surprised at how few calories you can eat, yet still feel completely satisfied. Do not snack between meals or after dinner. Never eat after dinner, as your stomach should be empty when you go to bed.

RAW FOOD VS COOKED FOOD

Some people may ask, "Why cook our foods?" You'll notice animals do not naturally eat cooked foods. Cooking our food is one thing that has given man freedom and independence. Fire is one of the four primordial elements (earth, wind, and water being the other three), and is basic to preparing our food. It seems to escape the advocates of a raw food diet that we're not animals, and aren't limited to raw foods. Cooking is necessary for such things as grains and beans. It does not kill enzymes. Heat transforms our food, and makes it more digestible. When you steam or lightly stir fry vegetables, they keep most all of their nutrition. Cooking is very yang, and changes the very nature of our food. If you look at people who have been on a raw food diet for any length of time, you'll see they are pale, weak, sickly, and have poor immunity and bad skin. Their choice of foods is also very limited. Nearly always, they are addicted to various sweets, and eat far too much dried fruit, fruit juice, tropical fruit, desserts, and sweeteners of various kinds. They are far too yin, which is reflected in their poor judgment and way of life. Cooking is a divine art, a sacred ceremony, and the kitchen is the center of the home. Use the magic of fire to change the very quality of your food.

FEEDING BABIES

What about babies? It is simply unbelievable that less than half the mothers in America choose to nurse their babies. The ones that don't are usually the same ones that choose C-section deliveries, in spite of the fact that the vast majority are able to nurse. We have lost touch with natural childbirth and child-feeding. Babies should be fed human milk, as this is obviously what is meant for them. If an acceptable wet nurse can be found, this will suffice. Under no circumstances should babies be fed cow or goat milk, which was meant for animals. These have such a different constitution as to be deleterious. If you cannot find human milk for your baby, feed it a combination of various grain and seed milks. Do *not* simply feed it soy milk, as this is too restrictive, and the isoflavone content would be excessive. Give your baby a variety of soy, rice, oat, flax, and almond milks. This is not as good as human milk, but will be nutritionally sound, and is infinitely better than cow or other animal milk. *The fact that two-thirds of Americans were weaned on cow milk is frightening.* The results of this are reflected in our present society, which is so far removed from harmony with natural laws. Clinical studies comparing people who were breast-fed to those raised on cow milk show better health, higher IQ, stronger immunity, and other benefits in the breast-fed ones. This is well documented in the published clinical literature.

EATING OUT

One important tenet of eating well is to avoid eating out as much as possible. Eat at home! Definitely take your lunch to work. Either eat breakfast at home and skip lunch, or take your own lunch. Take some food with you when you go out instead of buying it. The best places to eat are generally Asian restaurants, such as Thai, Korean, Chinese, Japanese, and Vietnamese. The ubiquitous white rice is not a problem, as you should only be doing this occasionally. However, some Asian restaurants now serve brown rice on request. Asian meals are your best choice overall. You'll find that whenever you go out to eat, you end up eating something you shouldn't and wouldn't be eating at home. Buffets such as Sizzler, Ryan's, and Golden Corral can be quite good, with a wide selection of various fresh vegetables and salads. Mexican restaurants offer vegetarian dishes, but ask that the cheese not be added to them. Indian restaurants have a tradition of vegetarianism, but avoid the dairy products. Vegetarian restaurants are usually only found in larger cities. You will find that major chains such as Subway, Applebee's, Ruby Tuesday, and other chains can offer healthy alternatives.

CONCLUSION

Japanese cooking is very healthy, but limited, restrictive, uncreative, and just not fun. This one cuisine has been the basis for macrobiotics, since the founders were Japanese. For over forty years, millions of people have limited themselves to this without questioning it. It is based on Japanese culture, and not the universal cuisines of the world. The traditional Japanese macrobiotic cookbooks are rather bland and uncreative. Go to your local library and get cookbooks from around the world. Use them to create interesting, varied, creative, and delicious meals, without watering down the health benefits of macrobiotics. Asian cookbooks are definitely the most promising and compatible with eating well. Chinese cuisine is generally the most creative and varied, and there are many different regional styles to choose from. Often you need make no changes at all in the recipes. Use the cuisines of the world to inspire you to eat whole healthy natural food in tune with the universal laws.

12. Calorie Restriction and Fasting

Americans are the fattest people on earth. Two-thirds of Americans are overweight or obese, and it gets worse every year. Obesity is an epidemic that now affects one-third of our children as well. What has happened in the last forty years? What has changed? If you look at any movie or television show filmed around 1970 or earlier, you don't see as many fat people. What has happened? What is different forty years later? The meat, potatoes, white bread, dairy, and sugar diet was as common then as it is now. However, today we eat twice the calories we need. We eat twice the protein we need. We eat eight times the fats we need. We are overfed and undernourished. It is not just that we eat too much, but now almost half the calories we eat are fat calories. We eat 42 percent fat calories, and most all of them artery-clogging, saturated animal fats. No one else eats this much fat. It isn't the food per se that makes you fat, but the fat you eat. *Eating fat makes you fat.*

The rural Chinese actually eat more calories than we do, but much more grains and vegetables, and far less meat, poultry, eggs, and dairy. They only eat about 15 percent fat calories, and mostly vegetable oils. They do far more physical work as well. We eat a mere 1 percent whole grains, when we should be eating at least 50 percent. Refined grains, empty calories, and the 160 pounds of sweeteners we eat every year all add to this. *Over 160 pounds of sugars per person yearly!* We never used to hog down sugar like this, and no other nation does it. Lack of exercise is certainly a factor. We are the richest nation on earth, have the least expensive and most abundant food supply and the highest standard of living materially. This affluence means we eat the most food per person and the most fat. As the American way of eating spreads into China and other Asian countries, their obesity rates and disease rates rise proportionately.

The United States spends much more on health care than any other country, yet we experience more illness and earlier deaths. We're the fattest nation on earth, and lead every other nation in most any disease rate. Obesity increases the risk of developing every known disease, lowers quality of life, and shortens our lifespan.

CALORIE RESTRICTION

You can eat as much as you want if you make better food choices. Diets don't work. They never have worked and never will work. *Just make better food choices.* The answer is making more intelligent, informed, and aware food choices. Just be in harmony with the universe that created and sustains us. You cannot go hungry for long, because the hunger instinct is too deeply imbedded for our very survival. Our desire to eat is actually much stronger than even our sexual instinct. You can go without sex your entire life, but it's hard to go without food for even a day. If you eat whole grains, beans, vegetables, seafood, salads, soups, and fruits, you can eat all you want and not be overweight. That's right, you can eat all the whole natural foods you want, never be hungry, and stay slim all your life. We eat twice the calories we need. A man only needs about 1,800 calories daily and a woman only about 1,200.

As mentioned in the previous chapter, the first thing you can do is stop eating three meals a day. We eat three meals a day, but only need two meals a day, regardless of the fact 99 percent of Americans eat three meals a day. This is one of the most basic and important changes to make in your life. Some people thrive on even less. Many Buddhist, Christian, and Hindu monks, for example, only eat one main meal. They may have a bowl of cereal in the morning, and then have their main meal in the evening. Would you rather skip breakfast or lunch? You can freely alter which meal you will skip daily. Many people will prefer to drop breakfast. They have so little time in the morning to prepare and eat food, since they are in a hurry to get to work. The less you eat, the better you'll feel, the healthier you will be, the fewer illnesses you will get, and the longer you'll live. Benjamin Franklin said, "To lengthen thy life, lessen thy meals."

The secret is not eating less food or going hungry. Just make better food choices. Consuming less calories slows the aging process, promotes healing, retards disease, and extends maximum lifespan. Glucose and insulin metabolism are improved, body temperature is lowered, immunity is enhanced, less illness and less severity of illness occurs, as well as less oxidative stress. Calorie restriction does not mean going hungry, but rather eating whole, natural, nutrient-dense foods that are low in fat and high in fiber and nutrition. More and more scientific evidence comes in every month, proving that calorie restriction is the single most powerful and effective means of extending our life span. That's right, calorie restriction beats everything else in effectiveness. *The less you eat, the longer you live.* Again, the average active woman only needs about 1,200 calories per day and the average active man only about 1,800 calories per day. Generally, we eat at least twice that here in America, and the results are all too obvious.

There has been quite a bit of research on the benefits of calorie restriction, especially on animals such as monkeys. It would take almost a century to fully study humans, but there has been a lot of shorter-term human research as well. The animal studies have shown this works best when started from birth. Calorie restriction still has dramatic benefits even when begun in middle or older age. It is never too late to start. Typical of this is a group effort done with the University of Wisconsin, Columbia University, and the Veterans Health Administration (*Toxicology Science* v. 52, 1999). Research on humans showed that people on calorie restriction for just a few years had much better health than the control group, and much better prospects for not only living longer, but suffering from less disease. There is no doubt about the effectiveness of calorie restriction. This is the most effective way to lengthen your life. With all this published research on calorie restriction, you would think there would be a good number of books and articles written on this subject. However, this isn't so. There only seems to be one author, Roy Walford, who wrote about calorie restriction (see Recommended Reading on page 107).

Calorie Density of Foods

This is how many pounds of each food a person would have to eat every day in order to get 2,500 calories. For example, you could only eat 10 ounces of vegetable oil at one extreme. On the other hand, you could eat 25 pounds of zucchini squash. You could eat a 15 ounce bag of almonds, or try to finish off 16 pounds of peaches. *The caloric intake would be the same.* The following listed grains and beans are cooked in the normal manner. Vegetables, fruits, seafood, poultry, and meat are raw. Values can vary here, but not much.

TABLE 12.1 CALORIE DENSITY (POUNDS CONSUMED)

DAIRY
Blue Cheese 1.5
Cream Cheese 1.5
Eggs (whole) 3.4

FATS
Butter 0.8
Vegetable Oil 0.6

FISH & SEAFOOD
Crab 5.9
Lobster 5.8
Mackerel 2.3
Salmon 3.9
Scallops 4.9
Shrimp 4.8
Tuna (in oil) 1.9
Tuna (in water) 4.3

FRUIT
Apples 9.4
Apricots 11.4
Bananas 6.4
Blackberries 9.4
Blueberries 8.8
Cantaloupe 18.2
Cherries 8.7
Coconut 1.6
Cranberries 12.4
Grapefruit 27.3
Grapes 11.9
Mangoes 8.3
Melons 18.2
Oranges 15.6
Peaches 16.6

Pears 9.0
Persimmon 19.5
Pineapple 10.5
Plums 9.1
Nectarines 9.3
Prunes 6.8
Pumpkin 16.6
Raspberries 7.5
Strawberries 14.8
Tangerines 16.1
Watermelon 21.0

GRAINS
Brown Rice 5.1
Buckwheat 5.9
Oatmeal 6.0
WW Pasta 3.1
WW Rolls 4.0

LEGUMES & BEANS
Black Beans 5.5
Chickpeas 4.6
Kidney Beans 5.6
Lentils 5.4
Millet 4.6
Navy Beans 4.8
Pink Beans 5.0
Pinto Beans 5.3

MEAT & POULTRY
Beef Chuck 1.4
Chicken 3.2
Ground Beef 1.9

Ham 2.1
Lamb Chops 2.2
Pork 2.1
Sirloin Steak 1.2
Turkey 2.1
Veal 3.4

NUTS & SEEDS
Almonds 0.9
Cashews 1.0
Chestnuts 3.5
Peanut Butter 0.9
Peanuts 0.9
Pistachios 0.9
Sesame Seeds 0.9
Walnuts 0.9

SNACKS
Cheez-Its 1.1
Chocolate Candy 1.0
Corn Chips 2.0
Potato Chips 2.0

SOY PRODUCTS
Soybeans 4.9
Soy Milk 10.1
Tofu 7.6

SWEETENERS
Honey 1.8
Sugar 1.5

VEGETABLES
Artichokes 26.0

Asparagus 21.0
Avocado 3.3
Beets 12.7
Brussels Sprouts 12.1
Cabbage 22.8
Carrots 13.0
Cauliflower 20.2
Celery 32.8
Collards 12.1
Corn 6.5
Cucumbers 32.8
Eggplant 28.8
Endive 27.3
French Fries 1.7
Green Beans 21.9
Green Peas 6.5
Lettuce 39.0
Mung Sprouts 15.6
Mushrooms 19.5
Mustard Greens 17.6
Okra 15.2
Olives 4.7
Onions 14.8
Potatoes 9.6
Radish 32.1
Seaweeds 12.4
Soy Sprouts 11.9
Spinach
Squash 28.8
Sweet Potato 5.4
Watercress 27.3
Yams 6.3
Zucchini 32.1

You can see that meat, dairy, poultry, and eggs have the highest calorie density because of their high fat content. Grains and beans are so low in calories that you can eat all you want. Fruits are very low in calories but can only be eaten in moderation because of their high sugar content. Green and yellow vegetables generally are lower in calories than any other food, and you can eat as many of these as you want. In fact, if you ate only fruit, or green and yellow vegetables, you couldn't get enough calories to live.

FASTING

Along with calorie restriction goes fasting. Fasting means water only; there is no other definition. People who speak of juice fasts really mean juice *feasts*. Such juice feasts are a total sugar overload. You can fast for a week very easily, and it is recommended for most people to do once a year. Heavy people can fast longer while using a vitamin and mineral supplement. As Christ said 2,000 years ago, when his disciples could not heal an afflicted man, "This kind goeth out not but by prayer and by fasting." The Old and New Testaments are full of references to fasting that are almost always ignored or explained away in modern churches. All religions have a long tradition of fasting, especially the Buddhists, Hindus, and Muslims. You don't have to be a religious person to fast, though, as fasting builds inner strength and character while healing, repairing, and cleansing the body. The wild animals know the value of fasting when they are sick or injured. Pythagoras, the philosopher, required his initiates to undergo a long fast before they could be accepted into his mystery school. This proved their character and sincerity.

The simplest and easiest way to start fasting is to choose one convenient day a week, then follow through fifty-two weeks a year. Every week, fast for one whole day, and this will become a most meaningful and enjoyable ritual for you. Eat your dinner, and do not eat again until dinner the next day. Normally one will simply be missing breakfast and lunch one day a week. Since you'll only be eating two meals a day, this would mean just missing one meal a day once a week. You can even do this very easily on vacations. If a special occasion comes up, just fast the day before or the day after. Always honor your weekly one-day fast, and never make excuses. This will give your body fifty-two days a year to rest, relax, purify, and repair itself. Just imagine fifty-two fasts a year! If you can't do this at first, just eat a bowl of hot soup instead of your first meal until you can fast. Our bodies are self-healing and self-repairing. Going without food for a period of time allows maximum healing and repair. The fifteenth-century physician Paracelsus said, "Fasting is the greatest remedy—the physician within." Take your supplements and hormones when you fast.

Surprisingly, feelings of hunger usually cease after the third day. Ironically, longer fasts can actually be easier, since there is little desire for food. At first, some people may experience mild side effects as toxins and poisons are expelled from their systems. The less side effects you experience, the healthier you are; the more side effects you experience, the more you need to fast. Headaches and a feeling of general sickness happen temporarily in some people, but these tend to go away quickly. Do not end your fast if you have side effects. Quite the contrary; this shows just how much you need to get these accumulated poisons out of your system. You will often feel happy, euphoric, clear headed, light, insightful, and energetic when you go without food. Fasting is very spiritually invigorating. There will be less physical strength, however. You can also fast two days every month. Just eat dinner and go without food until dinner two days later. For longer fasts, you can go to fasting centers by typing in "fasting centers" on your favorite Internet search engine. You can actually go two weeks without eating, especially if you are overweight. Fasting should be a regular part of your life for mental, physical, and spiritual strength.

For more information on fasting, see the Recommended Reading on page 107. Paul and Patricia Bragg are probably the best authors on fasting. You will find the dietary advice in the Recommended Reading books to differ from macrobiotics, however. Just read the books for the fasting advice.

CONCLUSION

Calories restriction is the most effective means of extending life known to science. Restricting your calorie intake can add years to your life. It will help you to experience weight loss, improve your health, and it could slow down the process of ageing. You do this by *making better food choices*, not going hungry. You should also fast weekly. Fasting is the most powerful healing method known. During a fast the body is detoxifying, healing, and repairing. Science shows that it also contributes to longer life expectancy.

13. Other Diets

Diet fads come and go with the times. That is just what these popular diets are—fads. In the 1960s, for example, the Scarsdale diet was the ultimate answer. With all the contradictory information and claims, how does one decide what really works and what doesn't? In one word: *results*. When you see people eating a certain way, are they healthy and happy? Are they slim and youthful? Do they look good and feel good? Are they vibrant and charismatic, with lots of energy and a good disposition? As the Bible tells us, "by their fruits shall ye know them." Look at the results of all these different ways of eating. Also look at the authors of these many different books. Most of these diet gurus are overweight, and have high cholesterol, blood pressure, and blood sugar. They look older than their years, despite plastic surgery. They suffer from a wide variety of illnesses they won't disclose. The whole grain-based way of eating we call macrobiotics is the only way that has been proven world-wide, over the decades, to result in maximum health. This is the only proven way to cure "incurable" illnesses, and no other way of eating can say that.

ATKINS DIET

The most popular diet in history is the ketogenic or Atkins diet. This high-fat, high-protein diet was proposed by Robert Atkins. It is now called the Paleolithic or Paleo diet. The argument is that this diet allows one to lose weight by using fat for energy. However, this forces the body to go into ketosis—a disease state characterized by excess blood ketones. The diet was named after a disease state! This is also a major cause of kidney disease.

Such a diet produces excess acetone, an especially toxic ketone, that gives people bad breath and body odor. Atkins died obese and sickly in 2003, at the age of only seventy-two. This was due to chronic coronary heart disease (cardiomyopathy) after following his own advice. He was the most popular diet author in history and sold more diet books than anyone else. This is proof that to be successful, you merely need to tell people what they want to hear. Atkins told people to eat all the meat, poultry, eggs, and dairy products they wanted to. Healthful whole grains like brown rice were completely forbidden. The most popular diet in history was completely backwards. The South Beach diet was a modification of the ketogenic diet, and soon failed as well.

BLOOD TYPE DIET

Another diet that has been popular for years is the one based on your blood type. Actually, your blood type has no relevance at all, except when you need a blood transfusion. Since people are always looking for a simplistic answer, this became surprisingly popular prior to its demise. The blood type diet says there are four basic blood types you should base your diet on. Type O means you are a Meat Eater, and should eat animal foods, but no whole grains or beans. Type A should eat a vegetarian diet and whole grains, but for some unexplained reason, the author just doesn't like wheat. Type B is the Nomad, and you can eat pretty much anything you want. This is the caveman diet, and dairy products are a staple. Type AB is the Enigma (only 5 percent of the population), and this combines the rules for both type A and B. How can such an irrational regimen become so popular?

BREATHITARIAN DIET

At the greatest extreme is the breathitarian diet. This advocates that you only eat raw fruits and nuts after they naturally fall off the tree. This is so you never hurt or kill anything. You begin by eating nothing but fruit and nuts, and eventually try to become so spiritual that you need no physical food at all. Instead, you live off of "prana," or cosmic energy. This is patently ridiculous, but they do have a point. Essentially, nothing in this universe exists but "sat-chit-ananda"—consciousness, energy, and bliss. *Food is nothing but manifested energy.* Theoretically, if you were enlightened, you would simply absorb universal, ever-present prana and not need physical food. This is nice in theory, but not in the real world.

FIT FOR LIFE DIET

One example of this raw food regimen was the food-combining, or Fit for Life diet. The concept suggests that when certain foods are mixed they are difficult to digest, and that a correct combination of foods should be practiced. This was based on the natural hygiene teachings of Herbert Shelton decades ago. Herbert died at age seventy-seven of Parkinson's disease, after following his own advice. This diet is based on eating fresh fruits, nuts, salads, and raw vegetables. There are numerous baseless rules, such as not combining starches with proteins and other prohibitions. The diet can quickly create serious nutritional deficiencies. Harvey Diamond temporarily revived this. Tony Robbins adopted it for years before admitting the diet just didn't work, and how poorly he and his wife had fared on such a regimen.

GLYCEMIC INDEX

This insanity is based on white bread as the Gold Standard! The central thesis is based on Wonder-type bread. The glycemic index claims to measure how much your blood sugar increases after eating a certain type of food. The problem is that this index is completely misleading. It doesn't even take into account the kind of carbohydrate consumed. The claim that whole grains raise blood sugar as much as candy bars, cakes, and pies is preposterous. All carbohydrates are somehow considered equal! The buzzword "carbs" is used constantly to refer to any and all carbohydrates. "Carbohydrate" is a meaningless term in that it refers to any food with carbon, hydrogen, and oxygen. Brown rice is considered biologically the same as white sugar, oatmeal the same as a Twinkies, and whole-grain bread no different than a candy bar. Many otherwise intelligent people have fallen for this transparent pseudoscience. You'll even see references to the glycemic index in scientific journals today.

MEDITERRANEAN DIET

The Mediterranean diet is still being promoted and is certainly better than the American or European diet. However, this is not nearly as healthy as most Asian diets. The Mediterranean diet incorporates white pasta, white bread, cheese, dairy foods, red meat, and far too much olive oil and tomatoes. Too many modifications have to be made here for this to be a basic style of eating.

VEGETARIAN
RAW FOOD DIET

Another popular diet is the vegetarian raw food diet. Here everything you eat must be raw and uncooked. This theory claims cooking is bad because it destroys the enzymes in "live food." The idea that cooking kills your food is plain silly. If a food doesn't taste good raw, you just don't eat it. Obviously, this limits most of your normal food choices. This is an overreaction to a lifetime of eating meat, poultry, eggs, and dairy products. People who eat this way very quickly become thin, weak, sickly, and suffer from bad skin and low immunity. Cooking grains and beans is necessary in order to eat them. Lightly cooking most of your green and yellow vegetables makes them more (not less) digestible and taste better. Certainly you should eat some raw foods and some salads with your meals—especially in warm climates, and in the summer. Just one month on a strict diet of raw, uncooked foods will quickly convince you that this is an irrational extreme which leads to debilitation. It is important to realize that cooking distinguishes us from animals, which are unable to cook their food. People who are ill often have difficulty in digesting raw foods, and do much better when their food is minimally cooked.

VEGETARIAN
AND VEGAN DIET

You can choose to be a pure vegetarian, or vegan. This simply means you omit seafood. Following a macrobiotic diet is therefore ideal for vegans. You'll find vegans to be more concerned about animal welfare than their health. So-called ovo-lacto vegetarians eat eggs, milk, and dairy products. Obviously, eggs and milk aren't vegetables. It is rather silly to call yourself a vegetarian when you eat them. Eggs, milk, and dairy are among the top ten allergenic foods known, and you can never be healthy eating this way. Many vegetarians and vegans are ethical by nature, and choose not to harm or exploit any animal life. This includes honey from bees, and anchovies in Worcestershire sauce. Such ideology is to be respected, but these people usually eat refined foods, tropical and nightshade foods, and inordinate amounts of various sugars. Many of them admit they are not eating for health, but only out of compassion for animals. Macrobiotics is a wonderful opportunity for people who want to be pure vegetarians to express their compassion while eating healthful, balanced, and nutritious food.

ZONE DIET

The Zone diet, or 30/30/40 plan, in which you control your zones of insulin values, fizzled after a few years. Barry Sears, the creator and promoter of the Zone diet, was obese and suffered from numerous health problems. This regimen includes lots of red meat, eggs, dairy products, poultry, white bread, and sugar. He recommended you eat a full 30 percent fat, especially saturated animal fat. This is four times what you need! He also recommended you eat 30 percent protein, which is at least twice what you need. This was obviously not a healthy way to live, despite its temporary popularity. One reason it became successful is that movie stars were following it. Now, that's certainly not a valid reason for choosing your diet! The theory was this overload of fat and protein would keep your insulin and glucose at proper levels for optimal blood sugar metabolism. The claims were made that you would achieve "superhealth," maintain lower insulin levels, lose fat, gain lean muscle mass, have more energy, lower cholesterol, and have better mental focus. Science, however, has proven that excess fat and protein are major causes of blood sugar dysmetabolism. Science has also demonstrated the best way to maintain optimum blood sugar levels is by eating whole grains.

CONCLUSION

No other diet has shown the results or stood the test of time like the whole-grain-based macrobiotic one. There are not many good diet authors. Susan Powter writes good books on eating well. Terry Shintani has actually published clinical studies on the benefits of a natural foods diet. The Pritikin diet has a lot going for it. Both Nathan Pritikin and his son Robert wrote basically good books. The Dean Ornish diet is a good low-fat diet, and includes a lot of whole grains. Neal Barnard has written good books on the vegan diet. Gary Null advocates a basically healthy diet. The John McDougall diet is pure vegetarian but includes too much sugar. All of these authors recommend nightshade vegetables and tropical foods. Surprisingly, none of them recommend proven supplements and natural hormone balance, much less fasting.

14. Natural Hormone Balance

Traditional Japanese macrobiotics does not use supplemental natural hormones for life extension. This is totally unreasonable. It is only in the last decade that such a wide variety of natural, bioidentical hormones have become inexpensively available over the counter, especially in the United States. Doctors rarely test patients for their hormone levels. Even endocrinologists are remarkably uninformed about testing and administering basic hormones. People who eat well, exercise, and live a healthy lifestyle do have somewhat better hormone profiles. However, this doesn't make up for the decline in our "good" hormones and the rise of our "bad" hormones as we age. The basic and most important ones to deal with are progesterone, estradiol, estrone, estriol, melatonin, testosterone, DHEA, pregnenolone, thyroid and growth hormones. Surprisingly, men and women both have exactly the same hormones, only in different amounts. Women have "male" testosterone, DHEA, and androstenedione, and men have "female" prolactin, LH, and FSH. Chapter 15 will tell you how to test these at home with saliva samples.

PROGESTERONE

Progesterone is important for both men and women. It is the antagonist to the powerful estrogens in our bodies, and balances the estradiol and estrone. Women are often prescribed unnatural oral progesterone analogs (chemical relatives) called progestins, instead of real, bioidentical, transdermal progesterone. Real progesterone is very poorly absorbed orally. Men have not been told how important progesterone is for their metabolism, or how it protects them from rising estrogen levels as they age. Women with PMS, menstrual irregularities, menopause, osteoporosis, arthritis, and other problems can benefit greatly from transdermal progesterone supplementation. Postmenopausal women can benefit the most from using progesterone, as their ovaries no longer produce it. Men over forty can benefit from using small amounts (i.e. a mere eighth of a teaspoon) of natural progesterone cream five days a week. This helps protect them from the current epidemic of prostate disorders. Progesterone is extremely safe and nontoxic, and has many proven benefits for both men and women.

Recommended Dosage: Buy a good two-ounce transdermal cream, with 1000 mg of real USP natural progesterone (500 mg per ounce).

ESTROGEN

Estrogen is a term that refers to the group of two dozen or so specific estrogens. Estradiol is the strongest, estrone second, and estriol very mild in comparison. Humans have 80 to 90 percent estriol, and 5 to 10 percent each of estrone and estradiol. Western women are rarely low in estradiol or estrone, contrary to the popular wisdom. Administering these hormones, especially those made from horse urine (Premarin), only makes their health worse, not better. Breast, cervical, uterine, and ovarian cancers are all basically caused by excessive unopposed (by progesterone) levels of estrogens. American women are generally plagued by excessive levels of estradiol and estrone from obesity, overeating, lack of exercise, high fat intake, drinking alcohol, and other causes. Estriol is the forgotten estrogen, even though it comprises 80 to 90 percent of human estrogen. Most Western women, especially those who are overweight, are low in estriol. It is not sold in regular pharmacies, and doctors are unfamiliar with it. Doctors who freely give women Premarin, estradiol, and estrone rarely even test women's blood levels before prescribing them. American women rarely test low in estrone and almost never in estradiol. Any estrogen must be used transdermally or sublingually. Never take oral forms of any estrogen, as they don't work. One-third of American women willingly consent to the surgical removal of their uterus at an average age of only thirty-five. This is surgical castration. It is somehow now considered normal and routine in America. The ovaries always atrophy and die afterwards, resulting in very serious hormone imbalance. Such women need overall hormone balance. *Men over fifty have higher estrogen levels than their menopausal wives!* This is a frightening fact and major reason men have a hormonal imbalance as they age. The only realistic way to lower excessive estrogen levels is to lose weight, eat a low-fat diet, exercise, avoid alcohol, and take proven supplements such as DIM and flax oil.

Recommended Dosage: You can buy a good 0.25 percent transdermal estriol cream (150 mg per 2-oz jar) on the Internet, or sublingual drops (500 mcg per drop) with a prescription.

DHEA

Dehydroepiandrosterone (DHEA) is a very powerful hormone, and our levels generally fall after the age of forty. Never take DHEA without first testing your blood or saliva level to see if you are deficient. Youthful levels are always the ideal, not high levels. Some people have excessive levels of DHEA. This is a pathological state, especially in women. Some men cannot metabolize oral DHEA (or any androgen) orally, transdermally, or sublingually, due to excess aromatase activity. Currently, there seems to be no answer for this. DHEA, or any androgen at all, simply turns into estradiol and estrone. There are several good books on the benefits of DHEA supplementation. The scientific literature is filled with literally thousands of studies proving the benefits of youthful levels as we age.

Recommended Dosage: If deficient, men can take about 25 mg and retest their levels after about three months. Women can take 12.5 mg (half-tablets) and should also retest after about three months. DHEA (like pregnenolone) is only about 10 percent absorbed orally.

MELATONIN

Melatonin is the most underrated of all hormones. The media tells you this is merely for better sleep and jet lag! Melatonin is critical for how long you live, how strong your immunity is, and how prone you are to getting such diseases as cancer. Good books have been written on melatonin if you want to learn more. The most impressive use is with cancer patients with a holistic program of diet, and balancing their other hormones. Melatonin levels fall in our teenage years and keep falling until we have very little left by the age of seventy. The most important benefit is extending our very lives. This is done by regulating our internal aging clocks. Mice given melatonin in their drinking water lived one-third longer than control mice. Imagine living to one hundred on the average rather than seventy-five, just by taking two dollars' worth of melatonin every month. Melatonin can be tested with saliva at 3:00 AM if you wish. This is extremely safe, without any known side effects, and scientists cannot even find an LD50 (lethal dose in 50 percent of test animals) for it. There is no such condition as naturally excessive melatonin levels, except in rare cases of pineal tumors. However, it would be very unsafe to exceed the youthful levels you had in your twenties.

Recommended Dosage: Three milligrams daily is a good general dose for men. Women can take half-tablets (1.5 mg). It is important to take melatonin only at night, as we do not produce this during the day.

TESTOSTERONE

Testosterone is important for both men and women, although men have about ten times more of it. Women can have naturally excessive levels, as they produce it in very different ways. Men cannot have naturally excessive levels. Testosterone falls in men after the age of forty. *Ninety percent of men are deficient by the age of fifty.* Women also generally decline, but can go either way as they age. It is ideal is to maintain the youthful level you had at the age of thirty. Women should look for midrange levels. You can use natural transdermal testosterone cream, DMSO solutions, or sublingual salts. It is important that you never use injected or oral testosterone. Men can use a 3 percent natural transdermal cream, which will deliver about 20 percent into the blood. A half-gram of this contains 15 mg, and will therefore get 3 mg into the blood. Men only make about 6 to 8 mg a day at age thirty. Women can use a weak 0.3 percent cream. A half gram of this contains 750 mcg (0.75 mg), and will therefore put about 150 mcg into the blood. Men can use 4 mg sublingual enanthate (which contains 3 mg testosterone), and women can use 200 mcg sublingual enanthate (containing 150 mg testosterone) from a compounding pharmacist. While women have one-tenth the amount of serum testosterone as men, they generally only need about one-twentieth the supplemental dose. This is because they metabolize testosterone more efficiently. Some men cannot metabolize any androgen, and therefore cannot use it.

Recommended Dosage: If women are deficient, they only need about 150 mcg in their blood every day. Men who are deficient need about 3 mg in their blood every day.

PREGNENOLONE

Pregnenolone is the "grandparent" hormone, since it produces all the other sex hormones. It is also the forgotten hormone, as it has been so little studied. It is incomprehensible why this basic hormone has been all but ignored ever since it was discovered. The studies we have are most impressive as to its importance. We do know that it is the most vital of all brain hormones, and very necessary for good cognition, memory, clear thought processes, and overall mental ability. Keeping youthful levels of pregnenolone will help you avoid senility and Alzheimer's as you age. Both men and women start losing pregnenolone at about the age of thirty-five. Pregnenolone (like DHEA) is only about 10 percent absorbed orally. Using pregnenolone with proven brain-friendly supplements like ALC, PS, and lecithin will help you have a strong mind all through your life.

Recommended Dosage: Men can take 50 mg daily, and women 25 mg, but you must retest after about three months. Adjust your dosage accordingly if necessary. You can get a blood test on the Internet without a doctor from www.labcorp.com.

CORTISOL

Cortisol is well named the stress hormone. Low cortisol is the ideal, while high cortisol generally indicates too much stress. To lower excessive corti- sol is not always easy, but can be done with diet, exercise, and lifestyle changes. If this is due to stress, you just cannot advise people to walk away from a bad marriage, change their profession, give their children away, escape from lifetime poverty, or whatever else is upsetting them. Exercise, meditation, sports, hobbies, owning a pet, and other such things can lower our cortisol levels. It is said that having higher DHEA and lower cortisol is a good indication of long life. You must do a comprehensive four-sample profile at, say, 9:00A.M./1:00P.M./5:00P.M./9:00P.M., since this varies so much during the day. You really don't need to bother with cortisol at all. It is what it is basically.

Recommended Dosage: Deficient levels are unusual, but can be raised with hydrocortisone (bioidentical cortisol), known as Cortef.

THYROID

Thyroid balance has been surprisingly neglected in life extension circles. Thyroid conditions, especially hypothyroidism, are epidemic in Americans over forty. You will get the most dramatic and demonstrable benefits from thyroid supplementation if you are deficient. Our thyroid secretes two hormones—T3 (triiodothyridine) and T4 (L-thyroxine). About 20 percent of this is T3 (which is four times stronger than T4), and about 80 percent is T4. You can get blood tests for free T3 and T4 levels on the Internet, without a doctor, by going to websites such as www.healthcheckusa.com. *You must be midrange, and not merely "in range."* Naturopathic doctors often recommend dried pig thyroid (Armour), which does contain the one-to-four ratio. The problem here is that people are rarely (maybe 5 percent) equally low in both

T3 and T4. Also, this is no more natural than the bioidentical T3 and T4 from the pharmacy. Excessive thyroid acitivity is much less common. If you have hyperthyroidism, do not resort to symptomatic harmful surgery, dangerous drugs, and outright deadly radiation to destroy thyroid tissue. Diet, lifestyle, and natural health practices are the real answer here.

Recommended Dosage: Bioidentical versions of both hormones are available as Cytomel/Cynomel, and Synthroid/Levoxyl. Buy the generic products. If you are shown to be low in T4, you would try 50 to 100 mcg to raise your level. If you are shown to be low in T3 you try one-fourth as much T3—12.5 to 25 mcg—since it is four times stronger.

GROWTH HORMONE (GH)

Our growth hormone (GH) levels fall from the time we are teenagers. They are extremely low by the age of seventy or so. Only in rare cases of acromegaly or pituitary tumors do we see excessive GH levels. You can get modest benefits from raising your growth hormone levels, especially if you are over sixty years of age. This just isn't worth the current price of having to inject it daily. Many people think this is a magic hormone merely because it is so expensive. The pharmaceutical companies could offer human growth hormone for $50 a month and still make a good profit, but they refuse to. Chinese GH, such as Hypertropin, is still pricey ($100 a month for 30 IU). American prescription growth hormone currently costs about $150 a month or more. This is supposed to be injected every day subcutaneously. You can use this sublingually in DMSO, but doctors cannot prescribe that. Oral and nasal secretagogues like hexarelin have all failed. Real world results are the best way to see the benefits. Like cortisol, you need a four-sample comprehensive profile. No matter what you hear, there are no oral, or over-the-counter supplements to raise your growth hormone levels. None of these have any value at all. Don't even think about using GH until all your other basic hormones are tested and balanced. You must balance all your other basic hormones first. Real human prescription GH has no more benefits than any other hormone. It is merely expensive and hard to manufacture a long 191-amino-acid chain. Meanwhile, keep your GH levels as high as possible with good diet, calorie restriction, weekly fasting, and lots of exercise—both aerobic and resistance.

Recommended Dosage: Balance all your other basic hormones, and use one gram of L-glutamine twice a day to temporarily spike your levels. You can also buy bulk glutamine and take one tablespoon a day. One I.U. a day of prescription GH is needed.

CONCLUSION

Our endocrine system is a harmonious balance, and all our hormones all work together as a team in concert. Raising one or two deficient hormones and ignoring the others has very little effect. Men and women need to balance their testosterone, DHEA, pregnenolone, melatonin, progesterone, T3, T4, and GH. Women need to balance their estradiol, estrone, and estriol as well. LH, FSH, and prolactin are optional. Men over forty would do well to test their estradiol and estrone to make sure they aren't excessive. Using natural hormones in natural ways along with blood or saliva testing, never has any negative side effects whatsoever. Hormone balance is central to good health and long life (one of the Seven Steps to Natural Health, see page 105).

15. Testing Your Hormones

It's very important for you test the levels of your basic hormones. Twenty years ago, the only way to test your hormone levels was to go to a specialist and order a very expensive blood analyses. Almost no one did this unless they had an unusual disease and were under the care of an endocrinologist. Even then, only a very few hormones would be tested, and at very high prices. Using a doctor to do this is still very expensive and unnecessary. The medical profession knows very little about natural hormone diagnosis or administration. That includes endocrinologists and gynecologists, as well as life-extension, holistic, and naturopathic doctors. There is almost no value in urinary hormone testing, as this only tells you how much of a hormone is excreted as waste. Anyone who advocates urine testing is clueless. Few doctors know that our sex hormones—especially testosterone, estradiol, and estrone—are mostly bound to sex hormone-binding globulin (SHBG), and are biologically unavailable. You want to test your free, unbound levels. Most doctors rarely test any hormone levels, and almost never test DHEA, pregnenolone, melatonin, estriol, or T3 and T4 levels. They are just not taught to in medical school.

HORMONE TESTS

There are much easier, cheaper, and less invasive ways to test your hormones (except growth hormone) without an unnecessary doctor's visit. They can be accurately tested at home with saliva, or with Internet blood testing services. For decades, clinics have used saliva instead of blood serum to test hormone levels. This is one of the greatest diagnostic breakthroughs of the last decade but is still relatively unknown. Now these can be done inexpensively at home without a prescription. Also, major labs now do blood testing online, without a doctor, for a wide range of hormones. Every year the list of which hormones they can analyze grows longer. The World Health Organization approved saliva testing in third world countries decades ago. You simply purchase a saliva kit, submit a saliva sample in a plastic tube, and mail it in a prepaid envelope to the laboratory. Sophisticated RIA (radioimmunoassay) testing accurately determines your hormone levels down to the very picogram (billionth of a gram). You will get a chart or table to show you the reference values for your age and sex so you can comprehend the results. All of this can be done for about $30 per hormone. The Internet blood testing sites refer you to clinics in a nearby city where a blood draw is done by a technician.

Ironically enough, you currently cannot find saliva testing kits in the drug stores, health food stores, or pharmacies. You must purchase them on the Internet. Type "in saliva hormone test," "hormone testing," or similar terms on your favorite search engine. If you are not on the Internet, just go down to your public library and ask the librarian to help you. Residents of New York, Maryland, and California need to use an out-of-state return address, as their legislators have made such testing illegal. This protects the salaries of the medical doctors. Even children, teenagers, and young adults can have hormone imbalances. These can only be detected by hormone testing.

Testing Progesterone Levels

Progesterone cannot be tested accurately with saliva, as it is oil soluble and must be serum (not plasma) tested. Women eighteen to forty can generally use progesterone without testing for it, since most of them have high estrogens, and many are anovulatory (do not produce eggs). Postmenopausal women can use progesterone without testing, since their ovaries no longer function. Any woman who does choose to test for progesterone must do so according to her menstrual cycle. Men don't need to test for progesterone at all. Men over forty can simply use it as discussed in the previous chapter.

Testing Estrogen Levels

All women over the age of thirteen would do well to test their three basic estrogens—estradiol (E2), estrone (E1), and estriol (E3). Hormone imbalance, especially with estrogens, is all too common among American women of all ages. These three can easily be tested according to your menstrual cycle. Western women are almost never low in estradiol, and rarely low in estrone. In fact, many of them have excessive levels of these two estrogens, especially those who are overweight. Western women are often deficient in estriol, especially if they are overweight. You want low normal values of E1 and E2. Healthy women, Asian women, and women who are vegetarians have lower levels of estradiol and estrone. Such women, however, have higher levels of estriol, so high normal values are the ideal. Men over forty can test their estradiol and estrone levels if they suspect estrogen dominance. Some indications are obesity, gynecomastia, and hair loss. Estriol imbalance in men is rare.

Testing DHEA Levels

DHEA can be saliva tested by men and women over forty, or younger people who feel hormone imbalance may be affecting them. Always look for youthful levels, and do not accept levels "normal for your age." Excessive or deficient levels can exist in people of any age, especially women. Men should be about 6.0 and women about 3.0 on the ZRT scale, since men have twice the level of DHEA as women.

Testing Melatonin Levels

Ideally, melatonin should be tested by anyone over the age of forty. You must do this at 3:00 AM with a saliva kit. (The only other alternative would be an expensive blood test from a sleep laboratory.) As we age, our melatonin levels almost disappear by the time we reach the age of seventy. Do not assume you are low just because you are over forty. Melatonin specific saliva kits are offered online. Women have half the blood level of melatonin as men.

Testing Testosterone Levels

Testosterone can easily be determined by saliva testing, and you will get the *free* testosterone results. Men over forty should test their testosterone levels. Women over forty, or women of any age who suspect high androgens, should test their testosterone levels as well. If you get a blood test, just insist that only your free testosterone be tested, and not the bound, or total testosterone. Doctors just don't test men for this, and feel women don't need to be tested! Men should be about 100 pg/ml and women should be about 30 pg/ml on the ZRT scale.

Testing Pregnenolone Levels

You can get a blood test for pregnenolone at Internet clinics such as www.healthcheckusa.com inexpensively, without a doctor. Pregnenolone saliva kits are not offered at the present time. Anyone over the age of forty should be able to safely take pregnenolone. This is the grandparent sex hormone, and all our other sex hormones are derived from it. Pregnenolone is also *the* most important brain and cognition hormone. Youthful pregnenolone levels will help prevent senility, memory loss, impaired cognition, and Alzheimer's in old age. Levels fall in both men and women after the age of thirty-five or forty, and then stabilize.

Testing Cortisol Levels

You can easily test your cortisol level, but it does vary from morning to night. There is no reason to get a blood test; use saliva testing. Do four tests four hours apart at, say, 9:00 AM, 1:00 PM, 5:00 PM, and 9:00 PM. This would give a good profile since cortisol varies so much during the day. This is very optional, and you don't need to test cortisol at all. It isn't practical to attempt to raise low cortisol levels. High levels can be lowered by diet and lifestyle.

Testing Thyroid Levels

It is very important you test your thyroid levels correctly. The medical profession will usually test your T3 uptake and TSH. The correct way to do this is to test your free T3 and free T4; any other thyroid parameter is optional. Doctors are generally misinformed and rarely test your actual free T3 and T4 levels. No saliva testing is offered at the present. If you see a doctor, insist that only your free T3 and free T4 be tested. A much better idea is to go to an Internet blood testing site such as www.healthcheckusa.com, where you do not need a doctor. You simply send them the money, they send you the paperwork, and you go to a member clinic in your area for a morning fasting blood draw by a technician.

Testing Growth Hormone Levels

Growth hormone is more problematic, since this is difficult to accurately test with a single blood draw. There are no saliva tests available at the present, but we will soon have saliva GH testing. Doctors or health advocates may tell you IGF-1 (which is easily tested by blood or saliva) accurately parallels growth hormone. It does not. If you are over fifty, you are most probably low in GH, and would modestly benefit from supplementation. To get a valid test you would need four blood draws in one day, four hours apart. A more practical way to determine this is to go by results rather than multiple blood draws. Just inject 1 IU of GH daily for 90 days, and go by real world results. Did your cholesterol and triglycerides fall? Did you lose body fat, and gain muscle mass (buy an inexpensive electronic impedence body fat scale for under $50)? Did you actually have more energy, sleep better, feel better, and not just imagine you did? Go by demonstrable results, and not placebo effects. Chinese GH costs about $1,200 a year, and should be injected. Sublingual GH in DMSO works, but cannot be prescribed by law. *Do not even consider this until all your other basic hormones are balanced.*

CONCLUSION

Stop depending on the medical profession for your diagnosis, since you can accurately and inexpensively do it yourself. Saliva hormone testing is one of the greatest medical breakthroughs in recent years, but you rarely hear anything about it. Now we also have the Internet to find blood testing available without a doctor. In California, Maryland, and New York, saliva testing is actually illegal! Internet blood testing is outlawed in states such as New Jersey. If you live in such states, just use a friend or relative in another state for your return address. More and more, we are going to see saliva testing popularized, and kits sold in drug stores and pharmacies. More and more, we are going to see Internet clinics offer blood testing without a doctor.

16. Natural Supplements

Traditional macrobiotics does not include natural supplements. Such blindness means you can never enjoy optimum health and longevity. It is only in the last decade that such a wide selection of vital nutritional supplements has become available. Understandably, this way of eating emphasizes that you get your nutrition from whole foods, rather than from supplements. This is correct. Eating whole natural foods does basically provide you with the nutrition you need. You should never look to compensate poor diet with nutritional supplements. *You simply cannot get all these vital factors from food.* Most people get their education on supplements from advertisers and promoters, and unfortunately they are very misled. In the last three decades, tremendous discoveries have been made in the area of life extension and natural health. Many medical journals now regularly include studies on natural supplements. Using this scientific technology in a sensible and holistic way will now allow us to heal illnesses faster, have stronger immunity, feel better, prevent disease, and live longer. We no longer have to rely on just the food we eat to be well. The simplistic idea of not using supplements just doesn't stand up at all to the light of reason or science.

ENDOGENOUS SUPPLEMENTS

Let's discuss some of the proven permanent natural endogenous supplements that we can benefit from. These supplements are found in your body and/or your normal foods.

Minerals and Trace Elements

Minerals and trace elements are deficient in most all people, no matter how well they eat. There are at least twenty-five elements we are known to need. We get enough potassium, sulfur, sodium, and phosphorous, which leaves at least twenty-one that should be supplemented. We are known to need magnesium, calcium, boron, vanadium, silicon, iron, selenium, chromium, iodine, molybdenum, zinc, manganese, tin, nickel, copper, germanium, strontium, cobalt, cesium, gallium, and rubidium. Search "mineral supplements" on Google to find one. None of the major vitamin companies offer more than ten of the above mentioned elements in the amounts you need. Search the Internet for "mineral supplements."

• Calcium must be addressed, since significant calcium is basically only found in dairy foods. The great majority of the world does not consume much, if any, dairy foods. People in Asia, Africa, and other areas generally don't eat dairy products. They take in far less calcium than we do, but have much better bone and joint health. Caucasians have the highest calcium intake on earth, yet the worst bone and joint health. The problem with calcium is not intake, but rather *absorption.* Remember that calcium cannot be absorbed without cofactors such as magnesium, boron, silicon, strontium, omega-3 fatty acids, and vitamin D.

Recommended Dosage: The official adult Recommended Dietary Allowance (RDA) of 1,000 mg is greatly exaggerated; 400 mg a day would certainly be sufficient. If you feel the need to take calcium supplements, take no more than 250 mg to 500 mg. Common forms such as citrates or carbonates are fine.

Multivitamins

Multivitamins are important no matter how well you eat. There are only thirteen known vitamins, and an RDA for each of them—A (5,000 IU), C (60 mg), D (400 IU), E (30 IU), K (80 mcg), B_1 (1.5 mg), B_2 (1.7 mg), niacin (20 mg), B_6 (2 mg), folic acid (400 mcg), biotin (300 mcg), pantothenic acid (10 mg), and B_{12} (2.4 mcg). It is very easy to find a multivitamin with all the vitamins you need in these RDAs. Be sure it has 1 mg (1,000 mcg) of methyl cobalamin, instead of regular vitamin B_{12}. Almost no vitamin supplements do this. Oral B_{12} is simply not absorbed well at all. Vitamin B_{12} is synthesized in our intestines based on the element cobalt. It is therefore important we get at least 25 mcg of cobalt every day. A popular pseudocriticism of vegetarian and macrobiotic diets is the supposed lack of vitamin B_{12}, since this is only found in animal foods. Is Nature so inept as to forget to put vitamin B$_{12}$ into plant foods? The countless millions of pure vegetarians in the world have never had a problem with this.

• **Beta carotene** is one of our most important antioxidants and is the direct precursor to vitamin A. The scientific validity of beta carotene supplementation has been extensively documented over the years. Include this in your regimen. It is a time-proven antioxidant.

Recommended Dosage: Take 10,000 IU in addition to the 5,000 IU of vitamin A you'll probably find in your daily vitamin tablet.

• **Vitamin C** has an RDA of only 60 mg, which you should find in your daily food. The macrobiotic diet has sometimes been criticized for the supposedly low amount of vitamin C. Vitamin C is extremely yin, and larger doses are only found in tropical fruits. You do not need a vitamin C supplement other than your multivitamin. People who take large doses (i.e. megadoses) debilitate their health and acidify their normally alkaline blood. Making your blood acidic lowers your immunity and ruins your health.

Recommended Dosage: You can take up to 250 mg if you want to, but no more.

• **Vitamin D** deficiency is epidemic in most countries. This is really a hormone, and not a vitamin. This is only found in some animal foods (like eggs) in very small amounts. It is not found in plant foods at all. Vitamin D is the most important and deficient of all thirteen vitamins. This is made by our skin on exposure to sunlight. Sickly and elderly people must take vitamin D. Never take more than 1,200 IU, as it is oil soluble, and builds up in the body.

Recommended Dosage: If you do not get regular exposure to the sun, it would be a good idea to take 400 IU a day in your multivitamin, plus an additional 400 to 800 IU, for a total of no more than 1,200 IU.

• **Vitamin E** is plentiful in whole grains, and you only need about 30 IU a day. This is very deficient since Americans only eat a mere one percent whole grains now. Taking an additional supplement of 200 IU (almost seven times the RDA) has been shown to have very strong benefits, especially for the cardiovascular system. The best type to take is the natural mixed tocopherols, instead of the cheaper single alpha-tocopherol. The research on vitamin E goes back decades and is well established in the medical literature.

Recommended Dosage: Take 200 IU daily. Higher doses will interfere with proper clotting. If you buy the popular 400 IU capsules, just take one every other day.

Acetyl-L-Carnitine

Acetyl-L-carnitine, or ALC, is more biologically available than plain L-carnitine. Studies prove the value of taking this for brain metabolism, memory, avoiding senility and Alzheimers, and general cognition. Use this along with pregnenolone, phosphatidylserine (PS), and even lecithin. This is a very important supplement.

Recommended Dosage: This is not expensive, and 500 mg a day should be enough for most people. Those over the age of sixty, or who are ill, can use 1,000 mg.

Acidophilus

Acidophilus with 6 billion or more units and 8 strains is very important for good digestion. Buy and keep it refrigerated, and use only reputable brands. Use this along with FOS and glutamine. There is also a stable spore form of acidophilus called LactoSpore, which you can take along with, or instead of, this. LactoSpore doesn't need refrigeration.

Recommended Dosage: Take one or two capsules daily of 6 billion units with 8 strains.

Beta Glucan

Beta glucan is the most powerful immune stimulant known to science, and not exotic, outrageously priced bioengineered interferon. This is an extract of yeast and mushrooms (1,3/1,6 configuration) or oats and barley (1,3/1,4 configuration). This has been known about for decades, but technology has not been able to inexpensively extract it until about the year 2000. Right now, the yeast-derived beta glucan is the strongest and least expensive. The yeast proteins are nearly all removed in the processing so you don't need to worry about yeast allergies. Don't take the overpriced mushroom extract or other preparations. Eating a small bowl of oatmeal or barley just three times a week will give you huge amounts, and you won't need a supplement.

Recommended Dosage: You can take 200 mg a day or 400 mg if you are elderly or ill.

Beta-sitosterols

Beta-sitosterols are in literally every vegetable you eat. This is an important supplement for both men and women. Find a brand with about 300 mg of mixed beta-sitosterols (with campesterol, stigmasterol, and brassicasterol). This is good for lowering cholesterol, and has shown preventative power in cancers, especially of the prostate, breast, and colon. Vegetarians get far more plant sterols in their diets than carnivores and omnivores. This is an excellent supplement to help prevent the epidemic of prostate and breast disease. Herbs like saw palmetto, pygeum, and nettles are useless because of their insignificant sterol content.

Recommended Dosage: You can take 600 mg if, you want, for one year. Then take 300 mg.

Carnosine

Carnosine is a fine supplement for heart health. Heart disease is the biggest killer of all. This is important for everyone over forty and those concerned with the health of their heart and arteries. There is good science here. Ironically, this is only found in meat, so vegetarians get none in their diet.

Recommended Dosage: Take 500 to 1,000 mg daily.

Coenzyme

Coenzyme Q_{10}, or CoQ_{10}, is a very important enzyme in our bodies, and supplementing this after the age of forty is very beneficial in many ways. As we age, the CoQ_{10} levels in organs like our hearts and brains fall severely. The research on this is stunning, especially for heart health, insulin regulation, healthy gums, and anti-cancer activity in general. Pay no more than $20 for 60 capsules of 100 mg. Insist on the real Japanese biocultured ubiquinone. *Do not take cheap unstable ubiquinol!* No reputable company will sell ubiquinol, as it has no shelf life. Be sure to take with flax oil or with food, as it is oil soluble. All "special delivery systems" are scams.

Recommended Dosage: You need 100 mg a day for it to do any good. If you are ill, or elderly, take 200 mg.

DIM

DIM, or diindolylmethane, is the direct metabolite of indole-3-carbinol or I3C. An extract of cruciferous vegetables (broccoli, cauliflower, and cabbage) called indole-3-carbinol (I3C) was discovered to have important anti-cancer properties. DIM lowers and improves the metabolism of estrogens in both men and women. Indole-3-carbinol breaks down to in our digestive system to DIM, which is twice as strong, and thus half the price. Find a 200 mg DIM supplement by surfing the Internet. This may be difficult to find in stores or catalogs at fair prices. Pay no more than $12 for 60 capsules of 200 mg each, and be sure not to take any less than this, as most all brands contain only 50 or 100 mg. Make sure to take with flax oil or food as it is oil soluble. All "special delivery systems" are scams.

Recommended Dosage: Take 200 mg each day.

Flax Oil

Flax oil is a much better source of omega-3 fatty acids than fish or krill oil for a variety of reasons. There are more omega-3s per gram, for one thing. Purchase your flax oil refrigerated and keep it refrigerated. We eat far too many omega-6 fatty acids, and far too little omega-3s, as there are so few good food sources of these. Valuable lignans are contained in high-lignan flax oil. It is less susceptible to oxidation than fish liver oils. Flax is the best source of omega-3 fatty acids known, and it is very difficult to get omega-3s, even on a macrobiotic diet.

Recommended Dosage: Taking one or two 1,000 mg softgels every day will go far to balance the ratio of omega-6 to omega-3 fatty acids in your system. You can also take one half-teaspoon of bulk (e.g. 12 oz) flax oil daily. You can grind flax seed every day, but this is impractical for most people.

FOS

FOS (fructooligosaccharides), otherwise known as insulin, is an indigestible sugar that feeds the good bacteria in your colon, but not the bad bacteria. It is important to keep your intestines strong and well balanced, as the digestive systems of Americans are generally in terrible shape. This is due to too many calories, too much fat, and too many toxins like excessive sweeteners, coffee and alcohol. Acidophilus, FOS, and L-glutamine, taken together, will do wonders for your intestinal health.

Recommended Dosage: Take one or two 750-mg capsules.

Glucosamine Sulfate

Glucosamine is an important building block in our joints and cartilage, but will not work alone. Glucosamine needs cofactors such as vitamins D, E and K, as well as sufficient minerals and trace elements, and flax oil. You should already be taking vitamins D and E. Vitamin K is the "forgotten vitamin," and you should be getting 80 mcg a day from your multivitamin. You should be getting the 20 minerals you need from your multimineral formula. Take flax oil as well.

Recommended Dosage: Take 500 to 1,000 mg a day for arthritis and rheumatism. Chondroitin is useless because the molecule is too large to pass through our intestinal walls.

Glutathione

Glutathione and SOD (superoxide dismutase) are the two most important antioxidant enzymes in our bodies. Taking glutathione is surprisingly not very effective for raising your levels. Taking 600 mg a day of NAC (N-acetyl cysteine) is a much more effective way to do this. Oral SOD is ineffective, nasal sprays are considered a prescription drug, and so far, no pharmaceutical company is interested in offering them. Oral SOD doesn't work. Currently, doctors are unaware of the dramatic benefits of SOD, and do not give injections. In the future, you'll see more nasal and injectable SOD products.

Recommended Dosage: Take 600 mg a day of NAC (N-acetyl cysteine).

Lecithin

Lecithin is phosphatidylcholine, and related to PS. Lecithin emulsifies fats. This is a proven, effective, and inexpensive supplement for good heart and artery health, normalizing cholesterol, helps preventing gallstones, supporting liver and bile metabolism, as well as good brain function. Lecithin contains choline, and has been studied for decades. It is extracted from soybeans. This is optional.

Recommended Dosage: You can take a 1,200 mg softgel every day.

L-glutamine

L-glutamine is another supplement to improve your intestinal health and help spike your growth hormone levels as well. This does not permanently raise your growth hormone level all day, but does spike blood GH for about two hours. Surgeons are actually giving patients L-glutamine after intestinal surgery to help them heal faster. You can also buy bulk glutamine and take a whole tablespoon a day.

Recommended Dosage: Take one gram of this inexpensive amino acid in the morning, and one gram before bed. This works very well with acidophilus and FOS.

Lipoic Acid

Lipoic acid is best known to help regulate our blood sugar metabolism. There are many other benefits such as brain function, cardiovascular health, liver function, and eyesight (especially glaucoma). Everyone over the age of forty should take lipoic acid for optimal health. This is not found in your food, but is manufactured by the body. Ignore false claims for the over-priced R-only form, as the clinical studies are all based on normal R-S lipoic acid. R-only lipoic acid is a scam, and you get 200 mg of R-only when you take 400 mg of regular lipoic acid (which is R,S lipoic acid).

Recommended Dosage: A good dose is 400 mg to insure proper blood sugar metabolism.

Phosphatidylserine

Phosphatidylserine, or PS, is an important chemical in our brains. This has been shown to be an important supplement for good cerebral function as we age. This is well worth $10 a month. PS has only become available in the last few years at a reasonable price. This is due to improved technology, and is now extracted from soybeans. The research is very impressive here. PS works best with ALC and pregnenolone. Also, 1,200 mg of lecithin can be added.

Recommended Dosage: You need 100 mg a day.

Quercetin

Quercetin is another natural and powerful antioxidant with clinical research behind it. Basically this is found in apples and the onion family. Quercetin is borderline endogenous and optional.

Recommended Dosage: Find an inexpensive 100 mg supplement, as we eat about 10 mg a day.

Soy Isoflavones

Soy isoflavones taken as a supplement is a much more realistic and practical way to get them. Most people just won't eat enough soy foods like soybeans, tofu, tempeh, and the like. Drinking a single glass of soymilk daily will add about 120 calories a day, or about 44,000 unnecessary calories a year, to your diet. These are not phytoestrogens, no matter what you have read—they are unrelated flavones, or plant pigments that have nothing whatsoever to do with estrogens. Estrogen of any kind is only found in animals and not in plants. The anti-soy hysteria is a product of the meat and dairy industry. Soy isoflavones are clinically proven worldwide in the published scientific literature.

Recommended Dosage: Taking a 40-mg soy isoflavone supplement is a better way to get the valuable benefits of daidzein and genistein.

EXOGENOUS SUPPLEMENTS

There are several temporary exogenous (not in your body or daily food) supplements you can take for about six months. Taking them any longer than this is a waste of money.

• **Aloe vera** is an old standard because it works. This is well known for topical use, but taking it internally can be good if you have poor digestion, stomach ulcers, or blood sugar dysmetabolism. It is also claimed to be good for immune enhancement. This can be considered a universal temporary supplement for everyone. Very concentrated 200-to-1 powdered extracts in capsules are now sold inexpensively. This makes it easier to take than spoonfuls of refrigerated gel. Aloe is time proven like lecithin.

Recommended Dosage: Take 100 to 200 mg of a good extract.

• **Citrus pectin** is a proven supplement to help lower cholesterol. Avoid the modified citrus pectin. Grapefruit or apple pectin is good.

Recommended Dosage: You must take 3 grams a day (6 x 500 mg capsules).

• **Curcumin** is an ancient Ayurvedic remedy known for thousands of years. There are good published clinical studies on this. This is a very powerful anti-inflammatory for arthritis and rheumatism, and a powerful antioxidant with potent anticancer properties.

Recommended Dosage: Find a supplement with 500 mg of actual curcuminoids.

• **Ellagic acid** is a powerful polyphenol antioxidant found in raspberry seeds, pomegranate, terminalia, and other plants. The actual amount of ellagic acid must be stated on the label, and not just how much extract of unstated purity.

Recommended Dosage: Taking 200 mg of this proven free radical fighter is a good idea, especially if you have an illness or condition of any kind.

• **Green tea** contains valuable antioxidant polyphenols, with many proven health benefits including anticancer activity. Green tea is just regular old tea before it is fermented to the common black tea. Therefore, green tea still contains caffeine. The same applies to bancha twig tea.

Recommended Dosage: Be sure to buy a decaffeinated extract.

• **Milk thistle** is the most proven and effective herb to promote good liver function, along with TMG. The science here is very good.

Recommended Dosage: Take two capsules daily of a reliable extract with high levels of silymarin, the active ingredient.

• **Sodium alginate** is a seaweed extract that removes toxic heavy metals, like mercury and lead, from your blood. Search the Internet for "sodium alginate."

Recommended Dosage: Take 3 grams a day for six to twelve months.

• **Trimethylglycine** (betaine), or TMG, is a proven supplement, but not well known. TMG is the most effective liver cleanser and rejuvenator known. It works well with milk thistle herb. If you have any liver problems, such as high SGOT or SGPT levels, non-alcoholic fatty liver, hepatitis, or inflammation, take this for one year. TMG also lowers homocysteine levels, which are a major indicator of heart health. Low homocysteine levels indicate longer life.

Recommended Dosage: Use 3 grams a day (6 X 500 mg) for six months to a year to help rejuvenate your liver. Then use one gram as maintenance.

• In addition to their daily vitamin, women over the age of forty should include **folic acid** and **vitamin B_6**. This would be in addition to their daily vitamin. The science on this is very impressive. Men do not need extra folic acid or B_6.

Recommended Dosage: Women over the age of forty should include an extra 400 to 800 mcg of folic acid and 10 mg of B_6. Do not exceed these doses.

CONCLUSION

In all these years of research, it has become obvious that many of the "wonder supplements" so heavily promoted simply have no scientific validation. Some of the most popular supplements currently sold do not have any clinical research behind them. The fact is, as consumers, we are subject to a constant barrage of commercial advertising promising instant cures, good health, and longer lives. Unfortunately, much of this isn't always true—in fact, many claims are exaggerated or just not true. The macrobiotic approach to life is based on decades of tried-and-true experiences. Every supplement in this chapter is verified by published, international, clinical research. It's best to take the supplements you know are proven to work in real human trials. If you are under forty, you should be taking about eight basic supplements—vitamins, minerals, beta glucan, vitamins D and E, flax oil, acidophilus, and FOS. You could add glutamine. If you are over forty, or have a serious health condition, you should be taking basically all of the above discussed permanent endogenous supplements, plus the hormones you need personally.

17. Meditation

When we refer to "zen macrobiotics," we are talking about meditation. Do you know what the word "zen" in Japanese means? It simply means meditation, just like "chan" does in Chinese. *Daily formal meditation should be the spiritual center of your life.* Without meditation there is no centering. Meditation is the door to spiritual illumination and freedom. A person who thinks all the time has nothing to think about but thoughts. We thus become disconnected from the reality of the world. There is no such thing as "deep thoughts" or "deep thinking." *All thought is shallow.* Reality is neither materialistic nor spiritual, nor both, nor neither. It is something that cannot be said, written, communicated, or described. If you can't say it, you can't sing it either. As J. Krishnamurti said, "There are no deep thoughts; all thoughts are shallow." The most difficult of all things is to have a silent mind beyond thought. Nothing is more difficult than this, as it is the door to enlightenment. In meditation, you are only concerned with the here and now. "Be here now" may be the best mantra of all. The past is a memory and the future a dream. When the knower becomes one with the known, you have reached enlightenment. An important tenet of Zen is "no purpose." How does one give up purpose except by having a purpose to give up? Paradox. There is only one Universal Ground of Being underlying all phenomena. In Hinduism, "sat-chit-ananda" means consciousness-energy-bliss. Nothing else exists but consciousness, energy, and bliss.

TECHNIQUES

There really are no meditation techniques, as this would clearly imply purposeful behavior. There is something you can do, though—simply watch your breath. No breathing techniques here—just silently watch your breath.

You'll see it is neither voluntary nor involuntary. Just quietly watch your breathing, and you'll notice it becomes deeper and stronger without any effort at all. Quite the contrary—if you make any effort it will not happen. An old Zen aphorism is, "If you strive, you fail; if you don't strive, you fail. What else is there?" After a while, you will take fewer breaths as you meditate. You will take just two or three breaths a minute, instead of a dozen. Why should you sit with your back straight up and your legs loosely crossed? This is actually the most comfortable way to sit for prolonged periods. Ideally, an hour of meditation a day is enough. This can be divided into half-hour morning and half-hour evening periods if you want.

If you have never read or heard of Alan Watts, he could be considered the premier American writer on Zen. The main book you should read by him is *The Book*. His other works are listed in the Recommended Reading section on page 107. There are also a variety of tapes, videos, and books edited after his death by his son, as well as a few books about Alan himself. D.T. Suzuki is another excellent author. Many audiobooks are now available as well. He is one of the finest writers on the Zen tradition ever. J. Krishnamurti wrote a variety of books. He is not the most entertaining. He comes off as rather serious, and his books can be somewhat dry. However, what he has to say will change your life, and leave no doubt about his enlightenment. If you want a real iconoclast, read Bhagwan Shree Rajneesh (aka Osho). The media hated him, and his ashrams were chaotic. The one thing he emphasized above all others is life has no meaning at all without meditation, without understanding who and what you are. He is very funny and unique, and criticizes everyone from Mother Teresa and the Pope to Mahatma Gandhi. He wrote dozens of books, and many of them are still available, as are the video tapes. You can't take yourself seriously anymore once you've read Osho.

CONCLUSION

Make meditation the most important part of your day, no matter how much time you put into it. Meditation will make you spiritually aware, center you, give you peace of mind, and illuminate your path in life. Our lives on earth are but brief flashes of light in the cosmos. We are only incarnated in physical form very temporarily. *Meditation is the only gate to see the universe as it is.* Without it we are empty.

18. Exercise

Surprisingly, traditional macrobiotics did not stress exercise. People in poor third world countries usually have to do manual labor and walk many miles a day just to stay alive. In the developed countries of the world, people actually have to go to swimming pools, gymnasiums, health clubs, tennis courts, golf courses, and other places to get any exercise. Unfortunately, most people in America just don't bother. Although you may enjoy skiing, tennis, soccer, basketball, softball, and other sports, you just aren't going to get regular year round workouts from these kinds of activities. You can choose aerobic exercise (the kind that makes you pant), or resistance exercise (weight training) or, ideally, a combination of both. You must enjoy your exercise sessions or you won't do them. Many runners have poor upper body strength, while many weight trainers have poor aerobic capacity. Most people have jobs, children, and endless responsibilities that leave little time or energy for exercise. Even walking the dog for a half hour becomes difficult. A third type of exercise is internal, and expressed in such disciplines as aikido, tai chi, and chi gong, which are meditative and spiritual in nature. These really do not give you the physical exercise you need, however. A combination of both aerobic exercise and resistance exercise is ideal.

BENEFITS OF EXERCISE

Physically fit people live longer than those who aren't. Exercise alone, with no other programs, can extend your lifespan up to five years. This has been demonstrated in multiple studies, including the famous Framingham Study, and the Harvard Alumni Health Study (*Journal of the American Medical Association* v. 273, 1995). It is never too late to start. It's not just about length of life, as important as that is. It is more about the combination of a long life with a high quality of life.

Diabetes

One in three American children will grow up diabetic. Diabetes and other blood sugar problems are a pandemic—not a mere epidemic—in people of all ages now. One of the basic reasons for this is our sedentary lifestyle. Real physical education classes should be emphasized in our schools, where the children really get a workout of some kind. Exercise lowers our blood sugar and insulin, and makes our cells more insulin sensitive. We have an epidemic of diabetes, metabolic syndrome, high blood sugar, and other associated problems that can all be prevented by sensible diet and lifestyle with lots of exercise.

Hormone Levels

Regular exercise is necessary to keep our hormonal system in balance. People who get regular exercise have much more youthful hormone levels, are healthier, feel better, and live longer. Studies around the world, including one by the University of Geneva (*International Journal of Sports Medicine* v. 18, 1997) prove this overwhelmingly. Exercise will help raise growth hormone, testosterone, DHEA, T3, and T4, while lowering estradiol, estrone, cortisol, and prolactin. In other words, being fit helps normalize and keep our entire endocrine system younger.

Coronary Heart Disease (CHD)

Physically fit people suffer from less heart and artery disease (the biggest killer by far), less cancer, less diabetes, less kidney and liver disease, less lung disease, and every other illness. You'll even sleep better! They have lower blood sugar, cholesterol, and triglycerides, C-reactive protein (CRP), homocysteine, and uric acid levels. (These are the six most important CHD diagnostics.) They have stronger immune systems, get less colds and the flu, and are less allergic. Exercise lowers oxidative stress and inflammation. This has been shown at such clinics as the University of Missouri (*Journal of Applied Physiology* v. 100, 2006). Oxidative stress is what ages us by excess free radical activity. Our two main antioxidant enzymes are superoxide dismutase (SOD) and glutathione. Both levels are higher in those who are physically conditioned. Inflammation is hard to define, but you can say it is redness, swelling, pain, tenderness, heat, and disturbed function in any area of the body. We suffer from very excessive oxidative stress and inflammation generally.

Hypertension

Hypertension is the most common medical condition in the world, affecting one-third of American adults, and one-half of those over sixty. Exercise is one of the best ways to lower blood pressure naturally. Sixty percent of all American adults are overweight, and now this affects children. One-third of all adults are outright obese. Exercise is necessary to stay slim all your life. This study shows all illness can be largely prevented simply by exercise.

Endorphins

There is a naturally occurring opiate neurotransmitter peptide in our bodies called beta-endorphin, which naturally makes us feel good. That's right, it is an opiate produced by the pituitary gland. Some call it endogenous morphine. Beta-endorphin levels go up dramatically during orgasm. People with higher levels of beta-endorphin actually feel better, rarely get depressed, don't get mood swings, suffer less illness, and live longer. They also tolerate pain better, as it is a natural analgesic. America leads the world in the use of prescription psychiatric drugs, especially for depression. Since those with high levels feel good, they are far less subject to alcohol and drug dependence. The best and easiest way to raise endorphins is by any kind of exercise, and preferably a combination of resistance and aerobic.

A massive study at UCLA (*Journal of Applied Physiology* v. 98, 2005) was complete with 424 references. *Effects of Exercise and Diet on Chronic Disease* demonstrates the importance of diet and exercise in our lives. Doctors Roberts and Barnard wisely bring up the point that an unhealthy diet and lack of exercise are really the leading cause of death in the world, since they are the very cause of the diseases we die from.

AEROBIC EXERCISE

Aerobic exercise is any moderate to intense activity that is done for an extended period of time. This raises your heart rate and oxygen absorption, and involves multiple muscle groups. In addition to strengthening your cardiovascular system, aerobic exercise improves immunity, reduces fatigue, and lowers your overall risk of illness.

Walking

The best overall exercise is simply walking briskly at a pace of about four miles an hour. Just a half-hour of walking a day will keep you in shape, but a whole hour would be ideal. *Walking will do wonders for you physically as well as mentally.* A daily walk will lower your blood pressure, help relieve stress, suppress appetite, help you lose weight (beyond merely burning calories), circulate your blood and improve blood parameters, stimulate digestion, relax you, help you sleep better, improve your appearance, help prevent coronary heart disease, lower your cholesterol, and regulate glucose metabolism. This will also give you a wonderful time to reflect on your life and deal with your everyday situations. Walking is miraculous! As stated by Thomas Jefferson, "The sovereign invigorator of the body is exercise, and of all the exercises walking is the best."

Jogging

Jogging and running are aerobic exercises, but most people don't find them as enjoyable as walking. Regular jogging, unlike walking, can have side effects such as shin splints, bone spurs, runner's knee (inflammation), foot stress mini-fractures, and swelling of the Achilles tendon. Be careful if you choose this.

RESISTANCE EXERCISE

Resistance exercise, or weight training, is for both men and women, especially ones over the age of thirty. Women gain strength and tone, while men gain strength and size. Doing fifty sets of weights twice a week is enough to keep anyone in top shape. Three times weekly is even better. One hundred sets a week can be done in less than an hour with circuit training. Circuit training is just doing one exercise after another, with only about fifteen seconds of resting between sets. You can ultimately learn to do fifty sets in just fifteen minutes this way, and spend only a half-hour a week at the gym. Circuit training is also aerobic.

The epidemic of osteoporosis, while prevalent among women, also affects a good number of men. It is very difficult to rebuild bone once it is lost, no matter how good your diet, supplement program, and hormone profile. It is far, far easier to prevent osteoporosis. As always, an ounce of prevention is worth ten pounds of cure. Resistance exercise stresses your bones, and tells them to be stronger. This is one reason poor people in third world countries have much stronger bones, and less bone and joint disease. They have to work hard physically, and put stress on their bones all throughout their lives. Safe resistance exercise will go a long way to help prevent and cure bone loss.

CONCLUSION

Exercise has to be a lifetime commitment, especially in our later years. Did you know that professional athletes such as runners, football, baseball, and basketball players actually live shorter lives and suffer from more ills than most of us on the average? One main reason is they only stay conditioned for a short period in their life, when they are young. This is not a lifelong fitness program for them. Another reason is most athletes eat high-protein, high-fat diets based on meat, poultry, eggs, and dairy products. You can never be slim, trim, fit, feel good, and stay youthful all your life without some kind of regular exercise. You simply have to exercise regularly. Admittedly, we live in a technological society where most of us work with our minds rather than our hands. Find the kind of exercise you enjoy, and stay with it the rest of your life. Physical fitness is priceless, and a cornerstone of good health.

19. Curing the Incurable

*Doctors are men who prescribe medicines of which they know little,
to cure diseases of which they know less, in human beings
of whom they know nothing.*
—VOLTAIRE

What is it that distinguishes the macrobiotic diet from the countless other diets that all claim to be the ideal, the best for us? What proof is there that eating whole grains, beans, and vegetables as our basic foods is really the ideal way of eating? Why should we put any faith in books such as this one? It's very simple. What other way of eating allows us to cure ourselves of "incurable" diseases, such as various cancers, diabetes, epilepsy, atherosclerosis, and others? Allopathic medicine only covers up the symptoms with palliatives. Remember that it is not diet per se that cures disease, but rather that our bodies cure themselves. Healthy diet allows our own healing powers to cure illness. It is common and everyday in macrobiotic circles to talk about people who have cured different kinds of cancer in less than a year. People with type 2 diabetes on medication can have normal blood sugar levels in six months. Men and women who were told they needed heart bypass surgery can clear their arteries in only a year. Men and women afflicted with epilepsy, on brain-deadening seizure medication, can be healthy and clear minded after a year or two of this lifestyle. *Macrobiotics works!*

CANCER

Every year cancer becomes more common. *Today, one in three Americans will end up with cancer before they die.* Nearly all American men over the age of seventy have prostate cancer. There will never be a medical cure for cancer. The real cure has always been getting in harmony with natural laws. The phony "war on cancer" has done nothing but waste money on allopathic studies, covering up the symptoms with radiation, surgery, and drugs. The cancer rates continue to rise, year after year. This is neither random nor caused by events beyond our control. Certainly there are minor genetic and environmental influences, but our diet and lifestyle are the basic causes. Diseases are a wake-up call from Nature for us to change our direction. This is not a "war" or a "fight" at all. When you are ill, Nature is telling you something is wrong, and you need to correct it. This is not some kind of battle at all, as we all are told. Americans eat twice the calories we need, five times the fat we need, twice the protein we need, and 160 pounds of various sugars we don't need at all. God knows how many toxic prescription drugs, and how much coffee, alcohol, and cigarettes we use. Add an endless variety of refined foods full of chemicals, preservatives, additives, and colorings we swill down. Then we wonder why we have such high rates of disease!

Case Studies

Everyone who has chosen to take this natural path should take the time to read some classic personal health books. If they are out of print, you can find them at your local library. These people did not have the advantage of the wide variety of effective supplements and natural hormones we are fortunate enough to have today. Also, they did not incorporate fasting in their healing regimen. Today we have all these things to help us get well.

Anthony Sattilaro was a medical doctor who was dying of prostate cancer. This is a relentless form that always ends in death. He, of course, doggedly believed in allopathic medicine. He turned his back on medicine, and simply changed his diet. His colleagues were appalled and shunned him. He cured himself within a year, and wrote the book *Recalled by Life* (see Recommended Reading list on page 107).

Milenka Dobic had stage IV ovarian cancer, which had already metastasized into her liver and lymph system. She was only given a few months to live. Milenka had a husband and daughter, and was just too young to die. She was ready to go through the usual surgery, radiation, and chemotherapy. Then she saw the women who had undergone this insanity, and was appalled! She saw the living hell they were suffering, and felt death would be preferable to being butchered, irradiated, and poisoned. Somehow, even in Yugoslavia, she found out about macrobiotics, and immediately changed her way of life. She and her family started eating whole grains, beans, and vegetables, instead of meat, chicken, potatoes, eggs, milk, and dairy products. Her health kept improving, and within two years she was cancer free. She wanted to share her experience with the world and so, in order to enlighten others as to the importance of macrobiotics, she wrote the book *My Beautiful Life*.

Dirk Benedict was a handsome, famous, rich, and happy actor who got prostate cancer in his thirties. He bravely decided he wanted to live, rather than be butchered, irradiated, and poisoned. In less than a year he was well and wrote *Confessions of a Kamikaze Cowboy*. He is now in his sixties, alive, youthful, happy, charismatic, creative, and the father of two handsome grown sons.

Elaine Nussbaum was a Jewish housewife who thought the sun rose and set on medical doctors. She allowed them to literally destroy her health and ravage her body when she got cancer. She was diagnosed with advanced uterine cancer, and given over twenty radiation treatments and implants. Her uterus and ovaries were removed. She was then given chemotherapy, and her vertebrae started to collapse. She became addicted to pain medication to the point that even morphine no longer stopped her suffering. She then got cancer of the spine and both lungs, and got ten more radiation treatments for a total of thirty exposures. She went on to more chemotherapy, and then to antibiotics and numerous blood transfusions, as she could no longer stop internal bleeding. She was now taking over three dozen pills a day. Near death and complete collapse, she changed her diet and lifestyle—and the entire course of her life. She was well within two years. She wrote *Recovery from Cancer* and she is now a dietary counselor to others.

There are many thousands of people who have read these books and cured themselves of all manner of "incurable" illnesses. They never wrote books and you'll never hear of them. Your author has been fortunate enough to work with men with prostate cancer for years now. These men just did not want to end up as the living dead, and intuitively knew there was a better way. Quality of life is what mattered to them, and not merely being technically alive and breathing. They chose to change their lifestyle and the food they ate. They first of all declined all medical treatments of any kind. They took the proven supplements and natural hormones. They exercised and even fasted for one day every week. All those who made any sincere attempt to cure themselves were well within about one year. The ones who didn't have the faith and character to change their lives went to the medical doctors. They all died after long periods of terrible suffering and expense.

DIABETES

Adult-onset diabetes is the leading health epidemic in the world today. One in three American children will grow up diabetic. All blood sugar dysfunction can be cured by eating a whole-grain-based diet. Have you noticed how uncommon diabetes is in rural Asia, Africa, and Latin America generally? If you are on diabetes medication, you can heal yourself, as long as you have an intact pancreas. The main cause of this is the inordinate intake of various sugars we have. Refined grains, high fat intake, obesity, and lack of exercise are other causes of this. As long as you have a viable pancreas, you can cure yourself in less than a year.

AIDS AND RADIATION POISONING

What "incurable" illness do you have? There is no reason you cannot heal yourself, and be well, if you truly want to live. However, there are two reservations that should be mentioned—AIDS and radiation poisoning. They are both manmade and not natural diseases. AIDS is the product of genetic bioengineering from military laboratories. HIV-positive people who have adopted a macrobiotic lifestyle went on to live their lives without progressing to AIDS. Once AIDS takes over you can live longer and better, but there is no cure. There is no concentrated radiation anywhere on the face of the earth, as this is a product of technology. Nathan Pritikin died of radiation-induced cancer despite a healthy diet and lots of exercise. He received extensive radium treatments when he was younger, which finally took their toll. He lived a much longer time with a far higher quality of life by following his own advice. The Pritikin diet was very close to macrobiotics. Once exposed to excessive doses of radiation, you can only mitigate the effects.

ALZHEIMER'S

Alzheimer's disease is something that can definitely be prevented by a macrobiotic lifestyle, but once it takes hold, there is no cure for it, either. The emphasis here is that it can be prevented, and you can be protected against ever coming down with it by following the principles of natural diet, proven supplements, and hormone balance. This is an illness that has only occurred in the last two centuries, basically, and was nonexistent before this. Alzheimer's is clearly different from common senility. The *Journal of the American Medical Association* (v. 265, 1991) revealed that Alzheimer's had increased a full thirteen times in the last ten years! A 1,300 percent increase in a decade. It has gotten worse since then. It is quite distinct from classic dementia. Aluminum intake is a factor, but the real cause is obvious—our declining diet and lifestyle.

ALLERGENIC FOODS

This is a good place to talk about allergenic foods. Milk and dairy products are the most allergenic foods, due to the lactose content, as well as the milk protein casein. The other top allergens are citrus fruit, chocolate, coffee, alcohol, poultry, strawberries, eggs, nightshade vegetables (potatoes, tomatoes, eggplants, and peppers), and peanuts. Any simple sugars, including all fruits, are not good for people with candida yeast syndrome. Unfortunately, a few people are allergic to fish and seafood. It is popular to say that wheat, corn, and soy are among the top allergens, but real world observation contradicts this. They are not. Gluten intolerance is another myth and is very rare. We just do not know how to accurately diagnose allergies. The current tests that claim to do so simply do not work, no matter what their assertions are. None of the current allergy diagnostic methods work. When we are able to diagnose which foods are compatible for each individual, a new day will dawn on natural medicine. Such diagnosis will also tell us which supplements and herbs will help us.

CONCLUSION

You can cure disease with a total program of diet and lifestyle. Diet is everything here. Follow the Seven Steps to Natural Health on page 105: diet, supplements, hormones, exercise, weekly fasting, no bad habits, and no drugs. It is not difficult to cure illness; the problem is the patient! Major conditions, like various cancers, coronary heart disease, diabetes, liver disease, kidney disease, lung disease, epilepsy, fibromyalgia, osteoporosis, can all be cured with diet and lifestyle. You are dealing with the very cause of your illness, rather than covering up the symptoms with drugs, surgery, radiation, and chemotherapy. Allopathic medicine just makes you worse in the end. Think holistic or whole body health. Treat your entire mind and body, and not just the condition you suffer from.

20. Caring For Your Pets

One-third of American families own dogs and cats. Are you feeding them healthy natural foods like the ones you eat? If you really love your pet, why are you feeding them that awful commercial pet food? Is it easier, more convenient, and cheaper? Feed them delicious, naturally healthy food they will enjoy. Animals cannot eat the same foods we eat because they have different digestive systems and teeth. Our pets have short digestive systems meant for digesting meat and animal foods, and teeth meant to rip and tear flesh. Carnivorism is their biological nature. Animals usually only eat once a day in the wild, and this is a good idea for domesticated ones. They are meant to eat meat and animal foods, and must have them to thrive. Fish and seafood can be a good staple especially for cats. Do not feed your pet milk and dairy foods as, like all the other animals, they do not eat these in their natural state. They are as lactose intolerant as we are. Eggs should be limited due to high fat and cholesterol content. Buddhist monks, for example, feed their temple cats a mixture of fish and whole grains, like barley and rice. They realize cats cannot exist on the same diet they eat. Misguided vegetarians try to feed their cats and dogs a vegetarian diet (usually with eggs and dairy products), which results in sickness and early death. Animals are meant to eat animal foods by nature.

COMMERCIAL PET FOOD

If you knew what was in commercial pet food you would never again feed this to your beloved friends. If you went to a pet food factory and saw the ingredients that are in them, you would never buy any again. Surprisingly, there are just no laws, rules, or regulations regarding pet food. Diseased animals, for example, are a main ingredient. Such things as tumors are allowed in the food. Most of these prepared foods have a high fat content. Commercial pet foods, no matter how well advertised, are not fit for your pet. This includes those expensive veterinary, refrigerated, and supposedly "natural" brands. It just takes a few minutes a day to feed your four-legged friends what you would want if you were them.

FOODS TO FEED YOUR PET

It really is quick, easy, and inexpensive to make your own pet food. You can make larger batches and freeze some of it. A good standard is to feed your pet half animal food and half whole grains, with a little green or yellow vegetable added. It is important to see they get some small amount of green or yellow vegetables for their vitamin A and other needs. They do eat this way in the wild, as they eat the stomachs and intestines of herbivores like rabbits and squirrels. This is one reason you'll see them eat grass. Again, do not feed them milk or dairy foods, as they do not eat these in the wild. It is very easy to find inexpensive cuts of pork, beef, chicken, turkey, various organ meats (like liver, kidneys, hearts, brains), fish, and shellfish. Do not choose fatty cuts. Many supermarkets have a section where short-dated meat is sold at half price. This is a great way to find inexpensive cuts of good pet food. Talk to the butcher about inexpensive types of meat and organs in bulk that can be frozen. Don't share any junk food or sweets, as this is not a real treat at all. If they are sick, let them go without food for a day or two as they would in the wild, as fasting is instinctual with them. Do not overfeed your dog or cat, and remember that calorie restriction works just as well in animals as in humans.

SUPPLEMENTS FOR YOUR PET

Your pets can also benefit greatly from many of the same supplements you use. Flax oil, acidophilus, FOS, multi-vitamins and minerals, beta glucan, and L-glutamine can be given to younger dogs and cats. NAC, lipoic acid, glucosamine, ALC, PS, CoQ_{10}, and carnosine can be added as they age. After middle age is when they really need these. Supplements like beta-sitosterol, beta carotene, soy isoflavones, quercetin, vitamin D, vitamin E, and DIM may not benefit animals. There is just no science here. There is almost no research done on pet health, diets, supplements, or hormones. It is important to understand that they should get amounts proportionate to their weight. A large 120-pound dog can take the same amounts of supplements you take. A 60-pound dogs can take half-doses. Small dogs and cats under 30 pounds can take quarter-doses.

TESTING YOUR PET'S HORMONE LEVELS

It would take a specialist to test the hormone levels of your cat or dog as they get older, and most people would not be willing to do this. Almost no veterinarians are versed in endocrinology. You can consider giving them melatonin, DHEA, pregnenolone, and progesterone cream when they get older. Males could get testosterone transdermally on their abdomen or inner ear. You might be able to have their thyroid tested. If you have had your male dog castrated, or your female dog's ovaries removed, they have a severe hormone imbalance and an equally severe biological imbalance from such destructive surgery.

EXERCISING YOUR PET

Be sure your dogs get a long walk at least once a day with you. This is their hunting time, and you are members of their pack. To them, you are pack members, and not masters or owners. Walking with you is more than just exercise—it is instinctual, and part of the bonding experience with their pack. Good food and exercise will prevent them from gaining weight.

BIRTH CONTROL FOR YOUR PET

The current castration for neutering and spaying dogs and cats is very harmful to your loving companion. This permanently unbalances their entire hormone system and impairs their health and well being. Yes, it is important to keep unwanted puppies from being born, but vasectomies and tubal ligations are much less harmful, practical, and less expensive means of doing this. This is what is used for humans. Would you cut castrate your son, or give your daughter a hysterectomy? You can find a vet who does these procedures as it is cheaper, easier, safer, and doesn't upset their hormone levels. Aren't your pets like children to you? *Do not castrate your pets!* Love your pets as you love your children.

CONCLUSION

Your pet should enjoy the same natural lifestyle you do. They are your family members. The most important thing is to make their food, and not give them commercial food. Give them the supplements they need. Walk them every day so you can bond with them as a pack. Many pets are kept at home and do not need birth control. If you need to do this, choose tubal ligation and vasectomy, not castration.

Seven Steps to Natural Health

The following steps are of vital importance for a long and healthy life. With these seven steps, you can prevent and treat "incurable" diseases like cancer, diabetes, heart disease, osteoporosis, arthritis, and others naturally, without drugs or invasive medical procedures like surgery and chemotherapy. You can also shed excess weight, fight obesity, and alleviate undesirable symptoms of menopause and premenstrual syndrome, all of which are affecting increasing numbers of women in the Western world. Every medical condition discussed in this book can be prevented, treated, or reversed with these seven essential steps. Along with stress reduction techniques like prayer and meditation, incorporate the guidelines below into your everyday life.

1. Follow an American macrobiotic whole grain-based diet. Diet is the single most crucial factor in achieving and maintaining good health. Diet prevents and cures disease. Everything else is secondary.

2. Take the proven nutritional supplements highlighted in Chapters 2 and 3 (see pages 8 to 17) to enhance the positive effects of your diet. Remember, if you are at least forty years of age, you should take all of the listed vitamins, minerals, and other nutrients.

3. Balance your hormone levels. If you are deficient in a certain hormone, take bioidentical hormone supplements. Excessive levels of a hormone can be lowered with diet and lifestyle. You can also easily and inexpensively measure your basic hormones using at-home saliva tests or an online lab.

4. Exercise regularly, even if you walk for just thirty minutes every day. Exercise is essential to your physical, mental, and emotional well-being. An ideal workout routine consists of both aerobic and resistance training.

5. Fast one day per week, drinking only water from dinner to dinner. Fasting is one of the most powerful healing methods known. You can also join Young Again's two-day fast, which takes place on the last weekend of every month. More information is available at www.youngagain.org.

6. Avoid prescription drugs. Exceptions are temporary antibiotics, pain medication in the event of an emergency, and necessary medications, such as insulin for type 1 diabetics.

7. End bad habits like drinking alcohol and using recreational drugs. You should also limit desserts and coffee consumption. You don't have to be a saint, but you do need to be responsible when it comes to matters of your health.

Recommended Reading

Adamson, Eve, and Linda Horning. *Complete Idiot's Guide to Fasting*. Indianapolis, IN: Amaranth, 2002.

Barnard, Neal. *Eat Right, Live Longer: Using the Natural Power of Foods to Age-Proof Your Body*. New York: Three Rivers Press, 2001.

—. *Food For Life: How the New Four Food Groups Can Save Your Life*. New York: Three Rivers Press, 1993.

—. *Live Longer, Live Better*. Summertown, TN: Book Publishing Company, 1999. (Audio.)

—. *Turn Off the Fat Genes: The Revolutionary Guide to Losing Weight*. New York: Three Rivers Press, 2001.

Benedict, Dirk. *Confessions of a Kamikaze Cowboy: A True Story of Discovery, Acting, Health, Illness, Recovery, and Life*. Garden City Park, NY: Square One Publishers, 2005.

Bragg, Patricia, and Paul C Bragg. *The Miracle of Fasting*. Santa Barbara, CA: Bragg Health Sciences, 2004.

Brown, Virginia, and Susan Stayman. *Macrobiotic Miracle: How a Vermont Family Overcame Cancer*. New York: Japan Publications, 1984.

Bueno-Aguer, Lee. *Fast Your Way to Health*. New Kensington, PA: Whitaker House, 1991.

Campbell, T. Colin, and Campbell, Thomas M. *The China Study*. Dallas, TX: BenBella Books, 2005.

Colbin, Annemarie, *The Natural Gourmet*. New York: Ballantine Books, 1989.

Cott, Allan. *Fasting: The Ultimate Diet*. Winter Park, FL: Hastings House, 2006.

Dobic, Mina. *My Beautiful Life: How I Conquered Cancer Naturally*. Garden City Park, NY: Square One Publishers, 2007.

Dufty, William. *Sugar Blues*. New York: Grand Central Life & Style, 1986.

Fuhrman, Joel, and Neal D Barnard. *Fasting and Eating for Health: A Medical Doctor's Program for Conquering Disease.* New York: St. Martin's Press, 1995.

Franklin, Jentezen. *The Fasting Edge.* Lake Mary, FL: Charisma House, 2011.

Kohler, Jean, and Alice Kohler. *Healing Miracles from Macrobiotics.* Upper Saddle River, NJ: Prentice Hall Trade, 1981.

Hellmiss, Margot, and Norbert Kriegisch. *Healthy Fasting.* New York: Sterling Publishing Company, 1999.

Krishnamurti, Jiddu. *Education and the Significance of Life.* New York, New York: HarperOne, 2008.

—. *The First and Last Freedom.* New York: Harper & Row, 1975.

—. *Freedom from the Known.* Edited by Mary Lutyens. New York: HarperSanFransisco, 2009.

—. *Meeting Life.* New York: HarperOne, 1991.

—. *Think on These Things.* New York: Harper & Row, 1981.

—.*This Light in Oneself.* Boston, MA: Shambhala Publication, Inc., 1999.

Kushi, Michio. *Standard Macrobiotic Diet.* Becket, MA: One Peaceful World Press, 1996.

—. *Your Body Never Lies: The Compete Book of Oriental Diagnosis.* Garden City Park, NY: Square One Publishers, 2006.

Kushi, Michio, Stephen Blauer, and Wendy Esko. *The Macrobiotic Way.* New York: Avery, 2004.

Kushi, Michio, and Edward Esko. *Macrobiotic Approach to Cancer.* New York: Avery, 1991.

Kushi, Michio, and Alex Jack. *The Book of Macrobiotics.* Garden City Park, NY: Square One Publishers, 2013.

—. *The Cancer Prevention Diet.* New York, New York: St. Martin's Press, 2009.

—. *Diet for a Strong Heart.* New York: St. Martin's Press, 2003.

Kushi, Michio and Aveline Kushi. *Macrobiotic Diet.* New York: Japan Publications, Inc., 1993.

McCarthy, Meredith. *Sweet and Natural: More Than 120 Sugar-Free Desserts.* New York: St. Martin's Press, 2001.

Null, Gary. *Get Healthy Now! A Complete Guide to Prevention, Treatment, and Healthy Living.* New York: Seven Stories Press, 2001.

—. *The Seven Steps to Perfect Health.* New York: ibooks, Inc., 2001.

—. *The Vegetarian Handbook: Eating Right for Total Health.* New York: St. Martin's Press, 1996.

Nussbaum, Elaine. *Recovery from Cancer.* Garden City Park, NY: Square One Publishers, 2003.

Ornish, Dean. *Eat More, Weigh Less: Dr. Dean Ornish's Life Choice Program for Losing Weight Safely While Eating Abundantly*, New York: Quill, 2001.

—. *Program for Reversing Heart Disease*. New York: Ballantine Books, 1996.

Nyoiti, Sakurazawa. *You Are All Sanpaku*. Translated by William Dufty. New York: Citadel Press, 2002.

Ohsawa, George. *Macrobiotics: The Way of Healing*. Chico, CA: George Ohsawa Macrobiotic Foundation, 1984.

—. *Zen Macrobiotics*. Chico, CA: George Ohsawa Macrobiotic Foundation, 1995.

Ohsawa, George, and Herman Aihara. *The Order of the Universe*. Chico, CA: George Oshawa Macrobiotic Foundation, 1986.

Ohsawa, George, and Carl Ferre. *Essential Ohsawa: From Food to Health, Happiness to Freedom*. Chico, CA: George Oshawa Macrobiotic Foundation, 2013.

Physicians Committee for Responsible Medicine. *Healthy Eating for Life for Women*. New York: John Wiley & Sons, Inc., 2002.

Pirello, Christina. *Christina Cooks: Everything You Always Wanted to Know About Whole Foods But Were Afraid to Ask*. New York: HPBooks, 2004.

—. *Cooking the Whole Foods Way: Your Complete, Everyday Guide to Healthy, Delicious Eating*. New York: HPBooks, 2007.

—. *Cook Your Way to the Life You Want*. New York: HPBooks, 1999.

Robert Pritikin. *The New Pritikin Program*. New York: Pocket Books, 2007.

—. *Pritikin Weight Loss Breakthrough: Five Easy Steps to Outsmart Your Fat Instinct*. New York: Signet, 1999.

—. *Pritikin Principle: The Calorie Density Solution*. New York: Time-Life Custom Publishing, 2000.

Powter, Susan. *Stop the Insanity*. New York: Pocket Books, 1993.

Robbins, John. *Healthy at 100*. New York: Ballantine Books, 2007.

Sattilaro, Anthony J., and Tom Monte. *Living Well Naturally*. Boston, MA: Houghton Mifflin Harcourt, 1985.

—. *Recalled by Life*. New York: HarperCollins, 1984.

Shelton, Herbert M. *Fasting for Renewal of Life*. Tampa, FL: National Health Association, 1974.

Shintani, Terry. *The Good Carbohydrate Revolution: A Proven Program for Low-Maintenance Weight Loss and Optimum Health*. New York: Pocket Books, 2002.

—. *The Hawaii Diet*. New York: Pocket Books, 1999.

Suzuki, D.T. *Zen Buddhism*. Edited by William Barrett. New York: Three Leaves Press, 2006.

—. *Zen Doctrine of No Mind*. Edited by Christmas Humphreys. York Beach, ME: Weiser Books, 1972.

Walford, Roy L. *Beyond the 120 Year Diet: How to Double Your Vital Years.* New York: Four Walls Eight Windows, 2000.

—. *Maximum Lifespan.* New York: W. W. Norton & Company, 2006.

Watts, Alan. *The Book: On the Taboo Against Knowing Who You Are.* New York: Vintage Books, 1989.

—. *Behold the Spirit: A Study in the Necessity of Mystical Religion.* New York: Vintage Books, 1972.

—. *Buddhism: The Religion of No-Religion.* Boston, MA: Tuttle Publishing, 1999.

— *Cloud-hidden, Whereabouts Unknown: A Mountain Journal.* New York: Vintage Books, 1974.

—. *Does It Matter? Essays on Man's Relation to Materiality.* Novato, CA: New World Library, 2007.

—. *In My Own Way: An Autobiography.* Novato, CA: New World Library, 2007.

—. *Myself: A Case of Mistaken Identity.* Louisville, CO: Sounds True, 2005. (Audio)

—. *Myth & Ritual in Christianity.* Charleston, SC: Nabu Press, 2011

—. *Nature, Man and Woman,* New York: Vintage Books, 1991.

—. *Psychotherapy East And West.* New York: Vintage Books, 1975.

—. *The Spirit of Zen: A Way of Life, Work, and Art in the Far East.* New York: Grove Press, 1994.

—. *Still the Mind: An Introduction to Meditation.* Novato, CA: New World Library, 2000.

—. *The Supreme Identity.* New York: Vintage Books, 1972.

—. *The Wisdom of Insecurity: A Message for an Age of Anxiety.* New York: Vintage Books, 2011.

—. *Tao: The Watercourse Way.* New York: Pantheon Books, 1975.

—. *This Is It, and Other Essays on Zen and Spiritual Experience.* New York: Vintage Books, 1973.

—. *The Two Hands of God: The Myths of Polarity.* Whitefish, MT: Literary Licensing LLC, 2011.

—. *What Is Tao?* Novato, CA: New World Library, 2000.

—. *What is Zen?* Novato, CA: New World Library, 2000.

—. *Zen and the Beat Way.* Boston, MA: Tuttle Publishing, 1997.

Willcox, Bradley. *The Okinawa Program.* New York: Three Rivers Press, 2002.

Williams, Dave. *Miracle Results of Fasting.* Tulsa, OK: Harrison House, 2005.

You can find all these books on www.amazon.com, or you can get them from your local public library, even if they are out of print. There are many other books on fasting.

About the Author

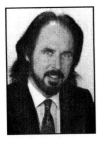

Roger Mason is an internationally known research chemist who studies natural health and life extension. He develops unique natural supplements and products. He writes books and articles, speaks to groups, and has a website. Roger has opened up a charitable trust, the Young Again Foundation, and continues to pursue his research in the many areas of natural health and healing. This is his tenth book on natural health. You can go to his website www.youngagain.org to get his free weekly newsletter and over three hundred articles on natural health. Roger and his wife live in Wilmington, NC.

Index